The Healing Dào
Chinese Medicine for Beginners

The Healing Dào
Chinese Medicine for Beginners

Achim Eckert, MD

World Scientific

NEW JERSEY • LONDON • SINGAPORE • BEIJING • SHANGHAI • HONG KONG • TAIPEI • CHENNAI • TOKYO

Published by

World Scientific Publishing Europe Ltd.
57 Shelton Street, Covent Garden, London WC2H 9HE
Head office: 5 Toh Tuck Link, Singapore 596224
USA office: 27 Warren Street, Suite 401-402, Hackensack, NJ 07601

Library of Congress Cataloging-in-Publication Data
Names: Eckert, Achim, author.
Title: The healing Dào : Chinese medicine for beginners / author Achim Eckert.
Description: New Jersey : World Scientific, [2025] | Includes bibliographical references and index.
Identifiers: LCCN 2024000545 | ISBN 9781800615380 (hardcover) |
    ISBN 9781800615519 (paperback) | ISBN 9781800615397 (ebook for institutions) |
    ISBN 9781800615403 (ebook for individuals)
Subjects: LCSH: Medicine, Chinese. | Taoist hygiene. | Mind and body therapies.
Classification: LCC R602 .E233 2025 | DDC 610.951--dc23/eng/20240202
LC record available at https://lccn.loc.gov/2024000545

British Library Cataloguing-in-Publication Data
A catalogue record for this book is available from the British Library.

Exercise photos: Stephan Huger (Vienna, Austria)
All other photos: Achim Eckert (Vienna, Austria)

Copyright © 2025 by Achim Eckert

All rights reserved.

For any available supplementary material, please visit
https://www.worldscientific.com/worldscibooks/10.1142/Q0455#t=suppl

Desk Editors: Nandha Kumar Krishnan/Rosie Williamson/Shi Ying Koe

Typeset by Stallion Press
Email: enquiries@stallionpress.com

About the Author

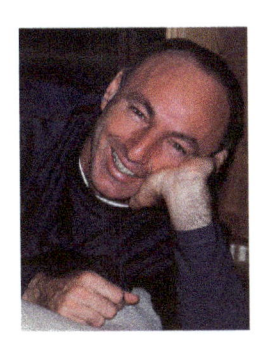

Achim Eckert was trained in Shiatsu, acupuncture, and Buddhist Meditation in Sri Lanka and India. To find ways to make acupuncture more efficient, he then studied structural fascia bodywork and body-oriented psychotherapy in California and Oregon. From 1992 to 1995, he headed a research project to investigate the psychological and psychosomatic effects of the 365 classical acupuncture points leading to the publication of *Das Tao der Akupressur und Akupunktur* (*The Dào of Acupressure and Acupuncture*) in Germany and *Acht Wundermeridiane* (*Eight Extraordinary Vessels*) in Austria. In 1996, he founded TAO Training as a synthesis of Shén Dào Fasciawork (to open up the meridians in the tissues), Traditional Chinese Medicine, and Reichian Bodywork. Since then he has been teaching this method in Germany, Austria, and Switzerland.

Readers can find a detailed description of his books in German, English, Spanish and Portuguese, as well as his seminar schedule in Germany, Austria and Brazil, at www.taotraining.at, contact: achim.eckert@gmx.at.

Contents

About the Author   v
Introduction   xi
First Steps to Chinese Medicine   xiii

Basic Concepts of Chinese Medicine   1
  Yin and Yáng   2
  The Chinese View of the Organs   7
  Zàng and Fu Organs   8
  Meridians   8
  Qì: The Life Force   10
  The Five Elements   11

Wood   15
  The Element Wood — Growth and Expansion   16
  Mental and Physical Exercises to Stimulate the
    Growth of Wood   30
    Clarifying questions   30
    Wood exercises   33
      Vision of the future   33
      Unexpressed anger   33
      Everyday irritation   34
      Movement   35
  Exercises for the Gallbladder and Liver Meridians   36
    Strengthening the Wood-Yáng   36
      The Gallbladder posture   36
      Activating the Gallbladder Meridian   38
    Strengthening the Wood-Yin   40
      The Liver posture   40
      Activating the Liver Meridian   41

Fire — 43
- The Element Fire — 44
- Mental and Physical Exercises to Ignite the Fire — 51
  - Clarifying questions — 51
  - Fire exercises — 52
    - Looking into the fire — 52
    - Light meditation — 53
    - Mirror meditation — 53
- Exercises for the Meridians of the Heart, Small Intestine, Pericardium, and San Jiao — 54
  - Strengthening the Fire-Yin — 54
    - The Heart posture — 54
    - Activating the Heart Meridian — 56
    - The Pericardium posture — 58
    - Activating the Pericardium — 59
  - Strengthening the Fire-Yáng — 60
    - The posture of the Small Intestine — 60
    - Activating the Small Intestine Meridian — 61
    - The San Jiao posture — 62
    - Activating the San Jiao — 63

Earth — 65
- The Element Earth — 66
- Mental and Physical Exercises to Strengthen the Earth — 75
  - Clarifying questions — 75
  - Earth exercises — 76
    - Grounding yourself — 76
    - Compassion — 77
    - Eating consciously — 77
- Exercises for the Stomach and Spleen Meridians — 78
  - Strengthening the Earth-Yáng — 78
    - The Stomach posture — 78
    - Activating the Stomach Meridian — 80

Strengthening the Earth-Yin	81
The Spleen posture	81
Activating the Spleen Meridian	83

Metal 85
The Element Metal	86
Mental and Physical Exercises to Refine Metal	92
Clarifying questions	92
Metal exercises	93
Rhythm of the breath and personality	93
Type I breather (tendency toward exhalation)	94
Type II breather (tendency toward inhalation)	95
Appreciating grief	96
Concentrating on what is important	96
Exercises for the Lung and Large Intestine Meridians	97
Strengthening the Metal-Yin	97
The Lung posture	97
Activating the Lung Meridian	98
Strengthening the Metal-Yáng	100
The Large Intestine posture	100
Activating the Large Intestine Meridian	101

Water 103
The Element Water	104
Mental and Physical Exercises to Get the Water Flowing	112
Clarifying questions	112
Water exercises	113
Confronting your fear	113
Feeling the womb	114
Latihan	115
Exercises for the Bladder and Kidney Meridians	116
Strengthening the Water-Yáng	116
The Bladder posture	116

Activating the Bladder Meridian: The candle and the plow	118
Strengthening the Water-Yin	120
The Kidney posture	120
Activating the Kidney Meridian	121

The Four Cycles — 123

The Shéng Cycle or the Law of Mother and Child	125
The Ko Cycle or the Law of Grandmother and Grandchild	129
The Cycle of Rebellion	136
The Cycle of Withdrawal	138
Practical Use of the Cycles	140

Epilogue — 143

The Dào of Healing in Times of War and Pandemic	149
Five-Element thinking	149
Chinese and Western allopathic medicine during the pandemic	157
Integrative medicine	159
TCM diagnostics	160
Qing Fei Pai Du Tang (QFPDD)	160
Chinese phytotherapy	161
TCM in the treatment of COVID-19 and Long COVID	162
TCM in Europe	163
Using TCM for prevention	164
The seven steps of healing	166
The year of the metal rat	171
Practical Solutions	174

Classification by the Five Elements — 177

Bibliography — 181

Index — 183

Introduction

In recent decades, there have been a number of notable changes as to how many people choose to live their lives. More and more people take the time to educate themselves about their health; they pay attention to nutrition, want to be physically fit, want to feel at home in their bodies, and try to understand what it is that makes them ill. Especially those with chronic illnesses indicate a preference for holistic methods of treatment, making use of methods, such as homeopathy, acupuncture, Chinese herbal, and Ayurveda treatments. At the same time, the psychosomatic aspects of illness are getting more and more attention, even among the proponents of evidence-based and technologically supported medicine. One sign of this transformation is an attempt to treat individuals more holistically: body, mind, and soul seen as an inseparable unit. This means that every physical illness at the same time denotes an underlying imbalance in the psyche or soul and must be treated accordingly.

This book was written from such an encompassing point of view — as a broad look at a world in which nature and humans are not separate — where philosophy and religion, psychology and medicine, and knowledge and wisdom go hand in hand. It takes a holistic understanding of people and our environment, health and disease, and body and soul.

First Steps to Chinese Medicine

My mother, who had studied literature and philosophy, introduced me to the great philosophers. At age 15, I was reading Hermann Hesse, Nietzsche, and Kant, and my heroes were Einstein, Gandhi, and Albert Schweitzer. My best friend and I sat in the park and dreamed about leaving school and going to India on a shoestring.

It was the time of the hippies, and the bus from London to Istanbul took three days, from Istanbul to Delhi a week, and from Delhi to Kathmandu another three days.

After school, aged 17, together with four friends I drove from Vienna, Austria, to India in a minibus. We left Vienna on June 10th 1974. Later I learned that this was the day of the first lecture of Bhagwan Shree Rajneesh, who would later become my teacher, in his new ashram in Pune.

One of us was the son of an Austrian diplomat, and thus we had some good addresses where to stay in Istanbul, Kabul, and Delhi. To save money, we slept in the car or just outside. No shower. Yugoslavia and Bulgaria were communist and an adventure. Bad roads. In Istanbul, the Austrian Embassy invited us to stay in a small castle at the Bosporus. It was an empty building but perfect for us to shower again and sleep on a mattress on a wooden floor for a couple of nights.

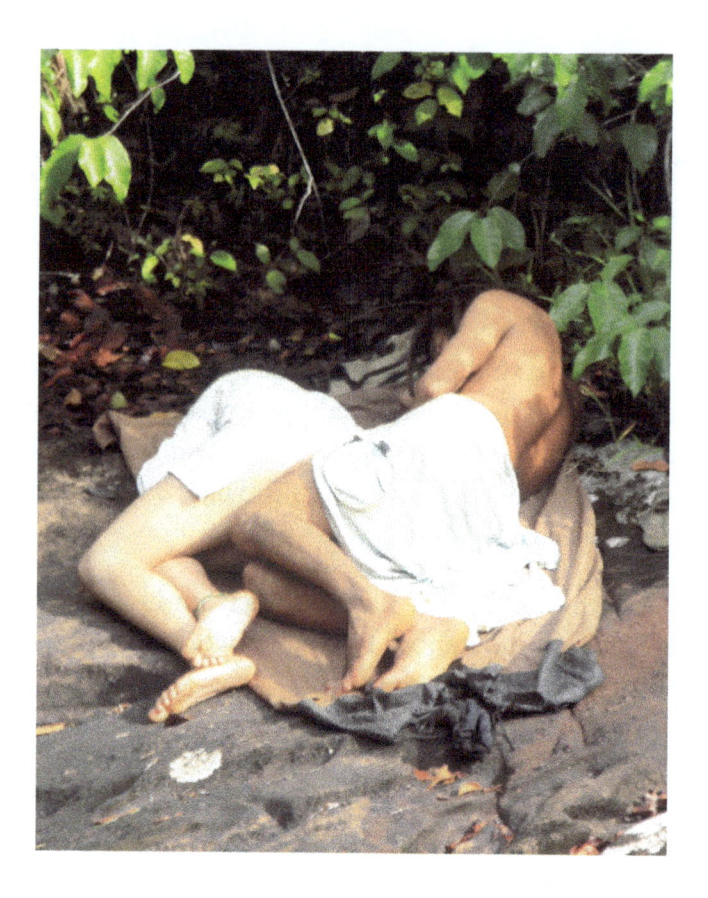

In Eastern Turkey, near Mount Ararat, we frequently encountered nomads who lived in tents. Today I think, they were Kurds. As we passed through their settlements, we were frequently offered bread and yogurt. I was not convinced that the yogurt was totally hygienic, but I didn't want to spurn their hospitality, so I didn't refuse. These people were the salt of the earth, simple and quiet.

Iran was very different. When we crossed the border at Maku, immediately we were surrounded by a group of young men wanting to buy a tape recorder or a camera, offering to trade it for hashish oil. No one bothered to roll a joint. The hashish oil was dropped on the cigarette from a small bottle — a simple procedure. Anyway, we needed the tape recorder and our two cameras and had nothing to trade.

We had the impression that many Iranians were quick-minded and business-oriented, and always some of us had to watch whether the petrol was put into the tank of the car or into some other vessel. It was during the reign of the Shah Rezah Pahlawi, four years before the Iranian Revolution in 1978. Women walked about in public without a veil. In Teheran, there were a lot of beautiful girls who caught our eyes.

Afghanistan was very different. Due to the summer heat, we often drove at night. In the villages we passed, the people slept on the street or beside their houses on the earth. Everyone felt safe to do so. Today, everybody is sleeping in houses that seem like small fortresses.

In any town we passed, the tables on the first fifty meters of every market were full of knives, swords, pistols, revolvers, guns, and Kalashnikovs. After the weapons came the rugs, clothes, fruit and vegetables, rice, beef, and lamb with a host of flies sitting on them. Many people lived in adobe houses with earthen floors. Houses that could afford a rug were considered palaces. Women were covered in black chadors, a veil that also covers the eyes.

The passes in the Hindukush often have an altitude of 3,000 meters or even higher. One was driving and the other four stood on the back bumper to jump off and push the van around the bends when the motor wasn't sufficiently ventilated.

We slept in the van, or just outside on the ground just covered with a blanket. All the shepherds in the area had a gun. But at that time, we felt safe, and we never encountered any violence.

In the valley of Bamiyan, we admired the Buddha statues that had been carved out of the rock. The tallest ones were 53 and 35 meters high. They originated from the sixth century and once upon a time used to be painted in lively colors; the hands and faces were ornamented with gems. The Islamic *conquista* of Afghanistan began in the eighth century. At that time, the population was mostly Buddhist or Hindu, some also Christian. In the following centuries, the statues were partly damaged by the Muslims, the gems were stolen and the genital areas destroyed. In 2001, the Taliban blew them up completely. It took them four days to destroy the massive rocks.

After three weeks in Afghanistan, we crossed the Khyber Pass to Pakistan. We spent some time in the tribal areas in the mountains of Pakistan, then visited the Golden Temple in Amritsar in India, and drove to Delhi. There I got bacterial dysentery with high fever and heavy diarrhoea. As I lost a lot of weight within 10 days, I flew back to Austria. Nevertheless, I had got a flavor of the Asian way of living and I would return there soon.

In Vienna, I began to study law and medicine. My personal motivation for studying medicine was to learn something about the functioning of my body in relation to my mind and vice versa. After studying medicine for three years at the University of Vienna, Austria, I felt that these studies were incomplete. Something was missing. Prior to this, I had had an old Chinese master who taught me Tài Ji and meditation. His name was Gia-Fu Feng. He had been the first to introduce me to the Chinese concept of Qì or Life Energy. During the same time, I participated in workshops on Reichian bodywork and Bioenergetics. My Reichian therapist talked about Orgone Energy — the Life Energy that Reich had discovered. And from lessons in a Yoga Ashram in Vienna I learned about Prana, the Hindu concept of Life Energy. Whether doing Bioenergetic exercises, Pranayama, or Tài Ji, the result was more or less the same: After a time of following the movements and exercises, I began to feel charged, my perception changed, and I felt happier and more alert.

So, I once again went to India to discover more about these sensations of happiness in my veins and the gradual changes of perception through all the Qì-enhancing exercises and meditation techniques that made colors look so brilliant, smells so overwhelming, and sounds so clear. I was looking for an Ashram and found one where I stayed for one and a half years. Thereupon I went to the Maldives on a kind of Robinson Crusoe trip, the only white person living on an island for about two months, eating bread, fruit, rice, and coconut, and watching a hundred kinds of fish. From there, I moved to Sri Lanka where I intended to set up a gem business to finance my further stay in Asia. One evening, while watching the sunset at the beach of Mount Lavinia, a coastal village south of Colombo, I became acquainted with three German doctors who had come to Sri Lanka to study acupuncture. They in turn introduced me to Prof. Sir Anton Jayasuriya who ran a governmentally financed acupuncture clinic in a country where most people were neither insured nor had money to pay for treatment when sick. I stayed in Sri Lanka for more than a year, working and studying at the acupuncture clinic of the Colombo South Hospital. At that time, we treated between 500 and 700 patients a day who arrived from all over the country usually after the rudimentary treatments with Western medicine and the devil dance of the village had failed. The treatment was free of charge, and sometimes we even gave them rupees for the bus fare and chai, the Sri Lankan version of spiced tea. During my time in Sri Lanka, I saw patients with a great variety of ailments: from asthma to elephantiasis, from epilepsy to paraplegia, from eczema to tinnitus, from glaucoma to high blood pressure, from stomatitis to gastric ulcers, and so forth. As the team consisted of an average of five doctors, there were lots of opportunities to learn about diagnosis and needling and to acquire a routine.

I remember the first day I arrived at the clinic. Prof Jayasuriya was treating a patient with acupuncture. One of the selected points was

Large Intestine 11, a point which is situated at the end of the elbow crease while the arm is flexed. With the next patient, he told me to put a needle into the same point. So I began to do acupuncture before actually knowing what I was doing. In the following weeks and months, I learned to do acupuncture more from a practical and empirical point of view, and it was difficult to keep studying the theory at night after work. Thus, I learned acupuncture from instinct rather than from knowledge, from the Heart rather than from the head.

During that year, there were not many students at the clinic. The German doctors had left, and for some months, there were two French students and a doctor from Melbourne. We rented a house on the beach together and experimented a lot with acupuncture and acupressure on ourselves and each other. I noticed that the needles, besides having an effect on my body and influencing my moods and emotions, also gradually altered my states of consciousness, that they broadened my perceptions, made my dreams more vivid and colorful, and helped to calm my mind so that I could be at ease and sit in meditation for hours on end.

In the following years, I had some other teachers of Traditional Chinese Medicine. I also learned Shiatsu and Chinese massage. I acquired most of these skills in India and Sri Lanka and, some years later, in California.

While working at the acupuncture clinic in Colombo, I asked myself why some people immediately responded to acupuncture and others did not. I observed that people who did physical labor responded better to acupuncture in general than people who did not move much. The flow of Qì obviously depended on the quality of the connective tissue in the body. As the commonly used acupuncture books were not precise about the exact location of the meridians in the body, I began to think of the meridians as tiny channels mostly running in the connective tissue between muscles and along major blood vessels and nerve chords, and the idea began to form in my mind that if it were possible to "open up" the tissue by massage, the effectiveness of acupuncture treatments could be enhanced considerably. Later, when I learned Postural Integration in California, a method of deep tissue structural bodywork similar to Rolfing and Rebalancing, this thesis proved to be true. After 10 or more sessions of deep tissue bodywork, I would do a thorough Chinese diagnosis according to the Five Elements. This would include Chinese pulse reading to ascertain the Fullness or Depletion of Qì in the various internal organs. Then I would use meridian massage to balance out Fullness and Depletion of Qì in the Twelve Organs and their corresponding meridians. And only if I could palpate a sufficient flow of Qì in the 12 Meridians, would I proceed to do acupuncture to guide the Qì to a place in the body, soul, and mind where it was needed — either because a symptom of a disease had remained in spite of all the bodywork and massage or to clear up a feeling and strengthen and enhance a physical, mental, or spiritual ability.

Although so many years have passed and I have encountered a multitude of philosophies and world views, my preferred system of thought for sorting things out and relating the varied phenomena of life to each other has remained the easily practicable Theory of the Five Elements. One of the main reasons for this is that it conclusively relates the material and spiritual world, the body, mind, and soul to each other. So far I have not found any other theory that is so handy and as, in the Western culture, medicine, and psychology, natural sciences and religion do not have a common frame of reference, I am really glad to have encountered this wonderful worldview and philosophy. After so many years I still teach the Theory of the Five Elements, Meridian Massage, and Shén Dào Fascia Bodywork which evolved as a synthesis of Deep Tissue Bodywork and Traditional Chinese Medicine — arranged in a way that the bodywork opens up the pathways of the meridians in the tissues, often between the muscles or along blood vessels and nerves. The result of Shén Dào Fascia Bodywork is an enhanced flow of Qì through the meridians that can be perceived as increased vitality and well-being and also be felt on the pulse.

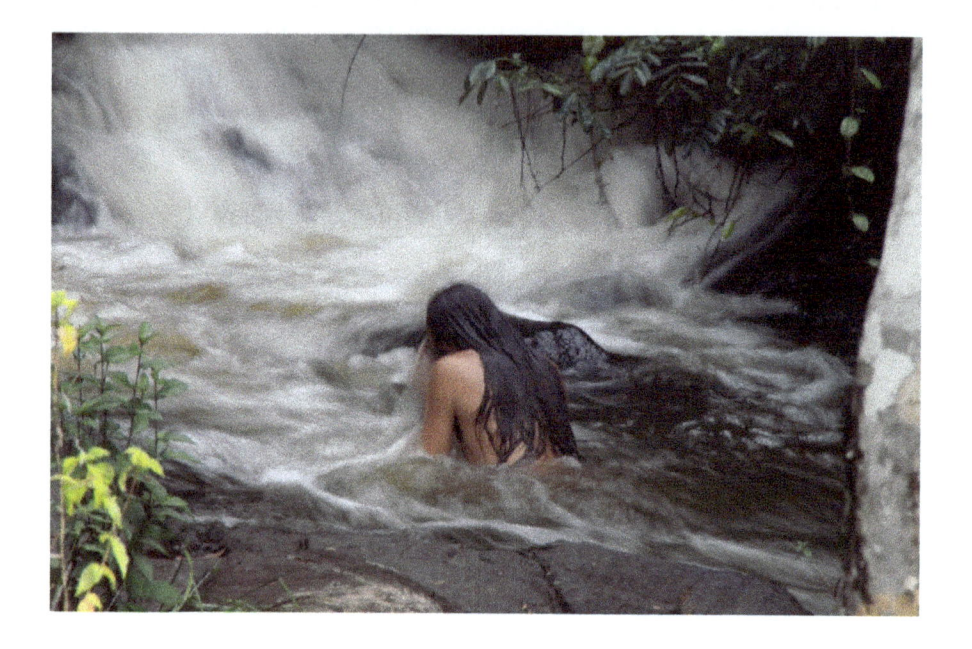

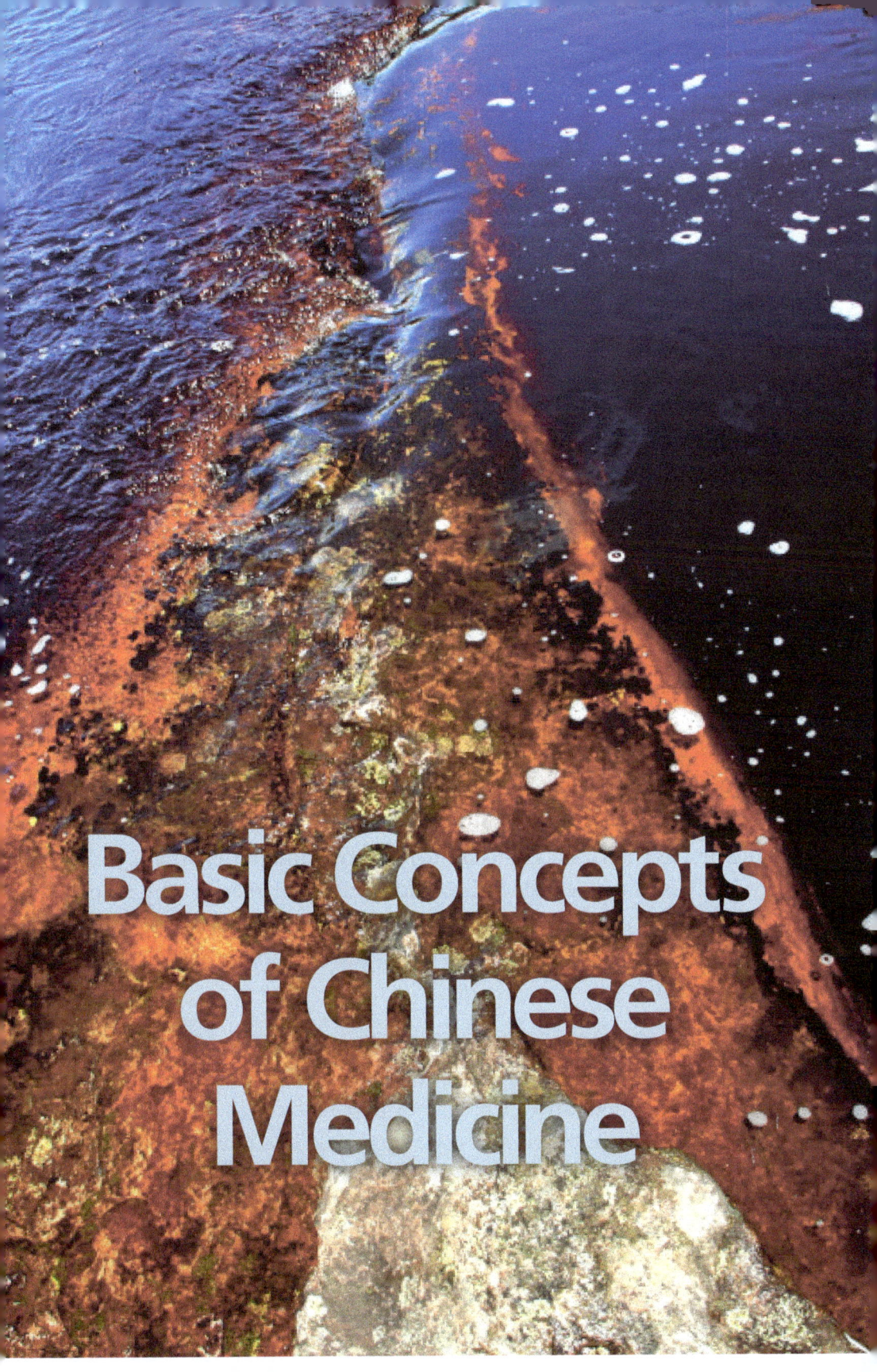

Basic Concepts of Chinese Medicine

Some of my readers might be familiar with the basic terminology of Chinese medicine, however, I would like to provide a brief introduction for those who do not have this background.

Yin and Yáng

Although these terms are widely known, they are frequently used in an imprecise way. One of the main reasons is that the Chinese and Japanese views on Yin and Yáng differ greatly. As many people nowadays might practice Shiatsu or Macrobiotics on the one hand, and on the other hand get Chinese herbal treatments and acupuncture, the notions of Yin and Yáng can become fuzzy at times.

The principle of Yin and Yáng is a Far Eastern way of seeing reality which conceives all different aspects of the world, material and spiritual, as being composed of two opposing and at the same time interdependent forces, namely Yin and Yáng. This dualistic thinking is not unknown to us. Occidental culture, Greek science, and philosophy, as well as Judeo-Christian religion are also built on the dual principle which we encounter in the concept of matter and energy in physics, in the ideas of good and bad and heaven and hell in Christian and Islamic religions, and in the binary code of our computer world. This could be a major reason why many aspects of Chinese and Japanese culture have been received more easily in the West than those from, for example, the Dogon in Central Africa.

However, it is important to understand that the Far Eastern concept of Yin and Yáng also differs from Western dualism. Yin and Yáng are opposites that form a whole; they depend on each other because they only exist in relation to their opposite. The Yin-Yáng symbol depicts the universal law of change. It tells us that one changes into the other at its extremes. The Yin and Yáng drop, each with a dot in the center of the opposite color, represents two poles which contain at their innermost core the essence of the opposite. In other words, nothing is merely Yin or Yáng, black or white, female or male, receptivity or giving, darkness or light, bad or good. This means that there are some male qualities in women and some female qualities in men, that there are always shades of gray, and that a "bad" action is never only "bad" and a "good" action may have "bad" consequences.

Yin and Yáng are no absolute terms. They are always used in a relative way, describing the relationships between the various phenomena of the material and spiritual world. To give you an example, in the body, the chest is viewed as Yin in comparison with the back, but in comparison with the pelvis, the chest is Yáng. Or another example, in comparison with day and daylight, the night is viewed as Yin, but in comparison with a black hole, our night on earth is Yáng because it still contains some light.

In Western culture, there is a tendency to take things that are relatives as absolutes. We have been educated to see things as either good or bad. But Yin and Yáng cannot be categorized as either good or bad. The Yin–Yáng symbol represents the way things change, it is a description, not a judgment. It tells us how opposites depend on each other, how they embrace each other, and how they finally become each other.

The following list of Yin and Yáng expresses the Chinese view and might differ considerably from the Japanese use of the terms. When using the list of Yin and Yáng, it is also important to remember the relative nature of the described opposites.

General Attributes

Yin	Yáng
Matter	Energy
Proton	Electron
Centripetal force	Centrifugal force
Consolidation	Expansion
Downward direction	Upward direction
Earth	Heaven
Horizontal	Vertical
Darkness	Light
Night	Day
Cold	Heat
Moon	Sun
Silver	Gold
Winter	Summer
End	Beginning
Old	Young
Negative	Positive
Passive	Active
Female	Male
Soft	Hard
In-flow	Out-flow
Rest	Movement
Slow	Fast
Interior	Exterior
Receptivity	Giving
Wet	Dry
Gravity	Growth
Roots, trunk	Branches, leaves
Fruit	Sprout, shoot
Alkaline	Acid

Body and Mind

Yin	Yáng
Front	Back
Left side	Right side
Lower body	Upper body
Trunk	Limbs
Legs	Arms
Pelvis	Head
Solid organs (*Zàng*)	Hollow organs (*Fu*)
Organs	Meridians
Yong Qì	*Wèi Qì*
Blood	Energy

Pathology

Yin	Yáng
Chronic	Acute
Internal diseases	Skin diseases and disorders of the sensory organs
Degenerative diseases	Infections
Pale face	Red face
Hypersalivation	Dry mouth
No thirst	Thirsty
Likes warm drink	Prefers cold drink
Cool body	Hot body
Oedema	Inflammation and fever
Slow and weak reactions	Fast and strong reactions to bacteria and viruses
Paralysis	Convulsions
Numbness	Spasms
Flaccidity	Cramps
Abundant menstruation	Scanty menstruation
Long menstrual cycle	Short menstrual cycle
Prefers quiet	Likes to move
Tiny voice	Loud voice
Moist skin	Dry skin
Puffy skin	Scaly skin
Diarrhoea	Constipation

Pain

Yin	Yáng
Chronic	Acute
Old	Recent
Permanent	Intermittent
Deep	Superficial
Diffuse, extended	Localized
Dull, heavy	Sharp, pulsating, itching, shooting
Worse by:	*Worse by:*
Nighttime	Daytime
Rest	Motion
Cold	Heat
Better by:	*Better by:*
Daytime	Nighttime
Motion	Rest
Heat	Cold
Soft touch	Firm pressure

Massage

Treating a Yin Condition	Treating a Yáng Condition
Gentle	Firm
Quick strokes	Slow strokes
Superficial	Deep
Upwards	Downward
Clockwise	Counterclockwise
Short duration (up to half an hour)	Long duration (an hour or more)
With the nails and fingertips	With the thumbs, palms, elbows, and feet

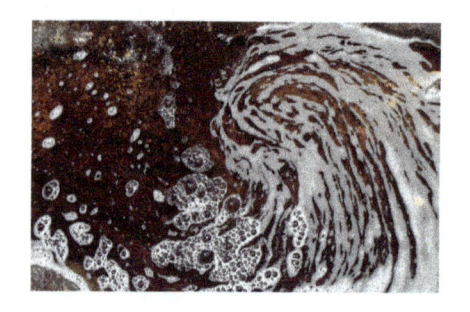

The Chinese View of the Organs

The Chinese view on the internal organs and body tissues quite differs from the Western concept. The reason is that Chinese culture does not separate body and soul. According to Chinese medicine, each organ has, in addition to its physical function, an emotional, mental, and spiritual function. Soul and mind are not just based in the Brain, rather in every cell in the body and in the entire energy field of the organism. The inner organs are interpreted more as a body-mind-spirit unit than as an anatomical form with physiological functions. Thus, each organ makes a contribution to the whole personality and its interactions with other organs are also of utmost importance on the mental and emotional levels.

As the organs are not looked upon from a merely physiological standpoint but from an elemental point of view that considers body, mind, and spirit as the expression of five elemental forces and their constant interplay, the anatomical definition of the various internal organs also differs from Western medicine. For example, the Stomach, the Duodenum, and the first six inches of the Small Intestine in Western terms are called the Stomach in Chinese medicine because the Chinese consider the digestive process and the absorption of nutrients from the digestive tract to the blood stream as the main task of the Earth Yáng organ: the Stomach. Another example, the Earth Yin organ, the Spleen, not only consists of the Spleen but also consists of the Pancreas and all the lymphatic tissue and organs in the body, the reason being that the duty of the Earth Yin organ, on the physical level, is to maintain the substance of the body. For this purpose, the Pancreas, which produces most of the digestive juices, as well as all the organs and cells, which constitute the immune system — such as Tonsils, Lymph Glands, and Spleen — are combined in one organ: the Spleen. To make a clear distinction between the Chinese and Western organ concepts, the organs, according to Chinese understanding, are spelled with capital initial letters in this book.

Zàng and Fu Organs

Chinese medicine differentiates between six Yin and six Yáng organs. The Yin organs are called Zàng: The character *Zàng* means firm or solid. The six Zàng have a firmer consistency than the six Fu. They are also called storage organs because, in addition to their physiological functions, they take up different forms of Qì and store, produce, or transform them. The six Zàng organs are the Heart, the Pericardium, the Liver, the Kidney, the Lung, and the Spleen.

The six Yáng organs are called Fu: The sign *fu* means hollow. The hollow organs are the Stomach, Small Intestine, Large Intestine, Gallbladder, Urinary Bladder, and Triple Warmer. The main tasks of the Fu are the reception and digestion of food, the absorption of nutrients, and the excretion of waste products. The duties of the Triple Warmer are the regulation of the temperature in the body and the coordination of the functions of the Chest, Abdomen, and Pelvis: the coordination of breathing, circulation, digestion, elimination, and sexuality.

Each Yáng organ is paired with a Fu organ of the same element. Their physiological, emotional, intellectual, and spiritual functions are closely related — each Zàng organ embodies the Yin power, and each Fu the Yáng force of the corresponding element.

Meridians

The channels that Qì, the life force or vital energy, flows through are the meridians, and the acupressure or acupuncture points are the places where you can tap into that energy flow.

Traditional Chinese medicine views the meridians as a network connecting the interior with the exterior: the internal organs with the surface of the body, tissue with spirit, Yin with Yáng, earth with sky.

It is a system of energy channels running mainly along the long axis of the body, with the exception of the Luò vessels and the Dai Mai, an extraordinary channel, which circles the waist like a belt. For this reason, it was compared by Western doctors to the meridian system of the earth: The organ meridians correspond with its longitudinal meridians, the Luò vessels with the latitudinal meridians, and the Dai Mai with the equator.

Already in the Huáng Dì Nèi Jing, the Yellow Emperor's Classic of Internal Medicine, which approximately dates back to the third century BCE, the pathway of the meridians and the effects of the acupuncture points are precisely and extensively described. In this text, the meridians are compared to the big rivers and streams of China which irrigate and fertilize the land. The Chinese character for meridian is *jing*, meaning river, path, track, or trail and, also, blood vessel.

The meridian system mainly consists of the 12 Organ Meridians, also called the 12 Regular Channels. Each of the 12 Organ Meridians pertains to and connects with a particular Zàng or Fu organ: The organ meridian is the main energy channel that connects the particular organ with other organs and the surface of the body.

The 12 Organ Meridians form pairs. Each Yin meridian is assigned to a Yáng meridian of the same element. These pairs are also called Coupled Meridians because their Qì flow is kept in balance by two sluice gates. These floodgates are the Luò vessels which form, together with the organ meridians, the network of channels that I mentioned above. Connecting the Coupled Meridians, their task is to ensure that the energy flow of Coupled Meridians is level, thus reducing the risk of an excess or deficiency of Qì in the particular meridian and its pertaining organ. The Chinese character *Luò* means to connect, to link, to tie together, and to network.

The function of the meridians and Luò vessels is to provide a circulation of Qì throughout the body, thus nourishing the tissues and linking up the whole body so as to keep the internal organs, four limbs, muscles, tendons, and bones intact and make the body an organic integrity.

Qì: The Life Force

Qì is the Chinese name for vital energy or Life Force. Its Japanese term is Ki, and in Yoga, it is called Prana. Most ancient cultures have the concept of an essential Life Force that circulates in the air, plants, animals, and the human body. It is the life behind the atom, the energy found in all forms of matter, and is concentrated in living organisms.

Although Paracelsus and Mesmer, healers of the sixteenth and eighteenth centuries in Europe, still used the notion of a Life Force, this term lost more and more importance over the course of Western medical history. Wilhelm Reich, an Austrian doctor who later emigrated to the USA, was the first to rediscover the vital energy or Life Force in scientific experiments in the twentieth century. He called it Orgone energy and had big problems with the FDA for manufacturing and selling Orgone accumulators, leading to his imprisonment and the public burning of his books in the USA in the fifties. During that time, the Russians also experimented with the Life Force, calling it Bioplasma. This led to the development of Kirlian photography with which it is possible to make the energy field of living organisms visible.

Already three to four thousand years ago, Indian and Chinese cultures developed systems of healing and meditation to enhance vital energy in people in order to prevent diseases and to heal the sick. The Chinese discerned various kinds of Life Force or Qì.

The most important terms for us to understand are Shí and Xu. Shí means Fullness or Excess of energy, leading mostly to Yáng or Hot symptoms, such as inflammation, pain, and fever. Xu means Depletion or Deficiency of energy, resulting mostly in Yin or Cold symptoms, such as chills, edema, numbness, and chronic pain. The meridian exercises which are described later in this book are used to balance out excess or deficiency of Qì in the various meridians and their corresponding organs, thus enhancing health and well-being.

The Chinese differentiated between acquired and congenital Qì. The congenital Qì that one inherits from one's parents and ancestors is therefore also called Ancestral Energy. The guardians of the Ancestral Energy are the Kidneys.

The Ancestral Energy is needed to form the Qì that one receives from food and air. In the Middle Warmer, Essential Energy, or Zong Qì, is "cooked" from food and air Qì, the Middle Warmer being the stove, the Ancestral Energy the fuel. The Zong Qì moves up to the chest, nourishes the Heart and Lungs to promote their functions, and divides into Yong Qì and Wèi Qì. Yong Qì is nutrient Qì; its function is to nourish the body and maintain its substance. Wèi Qì is defensive energy which defends the organism against exogenous pathogenic factors.

The Five Elements

In the Daoist teachings of the Five Elements, also referred to as "natural powers," the connections of the elements, the body, and the spirit are described in detail. These elements and the laws by which they operate can be observed at work in all natural phenomena, including the human being.

In Western culture, the laws of nature concerning the physical world are formulated. They are limited to things that can be measured physically, and they cannot be used in the realms of emotions and thought, fantasy, and intuition. As a result, our culture is often described as one-sided. As rich, precise, and varied as our knowledge of the material world may be, our knowledge of the psyche and the mental world is limited, confused, and speculative. Most of the time we are not even aware of how limited our thoughts are. Studying the *I Ching* (*The Book of Changes*) or the spiritual world of the Tibetan Lamas, Japanese Zen masters, or Native American shamans can show us that dimensions exist beyond the psychological and religious knowledge of Western culture.

In ancient China, the laws of nature were formulated so that the observed phenomena of both the material world and the spiritual world could be explained, and a relationship between them could be established. The separation into a material and nonmaterial world did not arise, at least not in our sense. At that time, the world was seen as an interplay of spirits and demons, of powers and forces of nature.

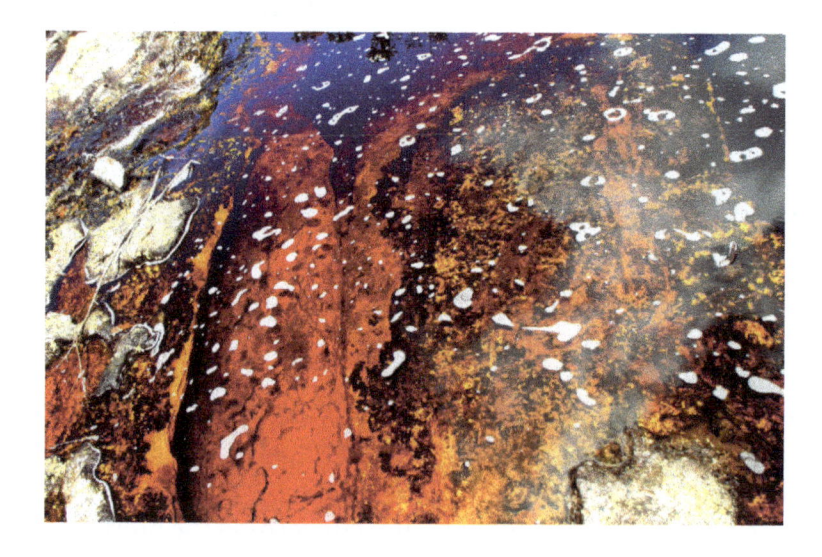

As in all cultures that are not "protected" by technology, ancient peoples both respected and feared the forces of nature: the drought bringing the heat of the summer, the typhoons, the tidal waves, and the rage of the gods in the thunder. It was common to call on the guardian spirits and to placate the demons. Earth, fire, heaven, and water were gods. One had to be aware of their signals if one wanted to survive.

These people began to observe and collect experiences, which they passed on from generation to generation. They observed the cycles of life, the courses of the stars, and the changes in weather; they observed these natural phenomena in connection with human beings, with their feelings and ways of thinking, with their dreams and their illnesses.

Out of these observations crystallized the teachings of the Dào. The Dào is also called "the unnameable" — that from which everything is born, yet that which has no direction, no will, no goal: that which is. The polarities are born out of the Dào: Yin and Yáng, earth and heaven, matter and energy. The Five Elements are born from Yin and Yáng. In their image, they bring forth, create, maintain, and break down the world.

It is important to understand that our term "element" does not have the same meaning as the Chinese term. The Chinese see an element not as a material substance but rather as a power, a specific quality of the universe. As the translation shows, this term is not limited to the power of nature but refers in general to its laws and principles. The elements are seen as transition phases of the varied manifestations, as energetic states that return again and again. The Chinese idea of transition phases and energetic states corresponds to modern discoveries in physics in an amazing way, especially to the idea of energy fields, quantum mechanics, and the Heisenberg

Uncertainty Principle. Scientists such as Niels Bohr and Fritjof Capra have recognized the similarity between quantum physics and Daoist worldview (see *The Tao of Physics* by Capra for details).

According to Chinese views, the Five Elements are evident in all manifestations in the cosmos: in the directions, the seasons, the climate, the stars, the plants and animals, the mineral and rock layers, and human beings. The senses, organs, and tissues of living beings are assigned to elements, as are emotions and mental abilities. The elements are powers that keep each other balanced; they create each other; they change into and block one another. If the energetic relationships of the elements are not balanced, this expresses itself in a human being as discomfort and illness, and in a society as weakness, injustice, and war. If the elements in a person — as well as in a society or a state — are balanced and strong, one finds harmony and health, beauty and grace.

In reading about the Five Elements, it may be helpful to refer to the chart "Classification by the Five Elements" at the back of this book.

Wood 木

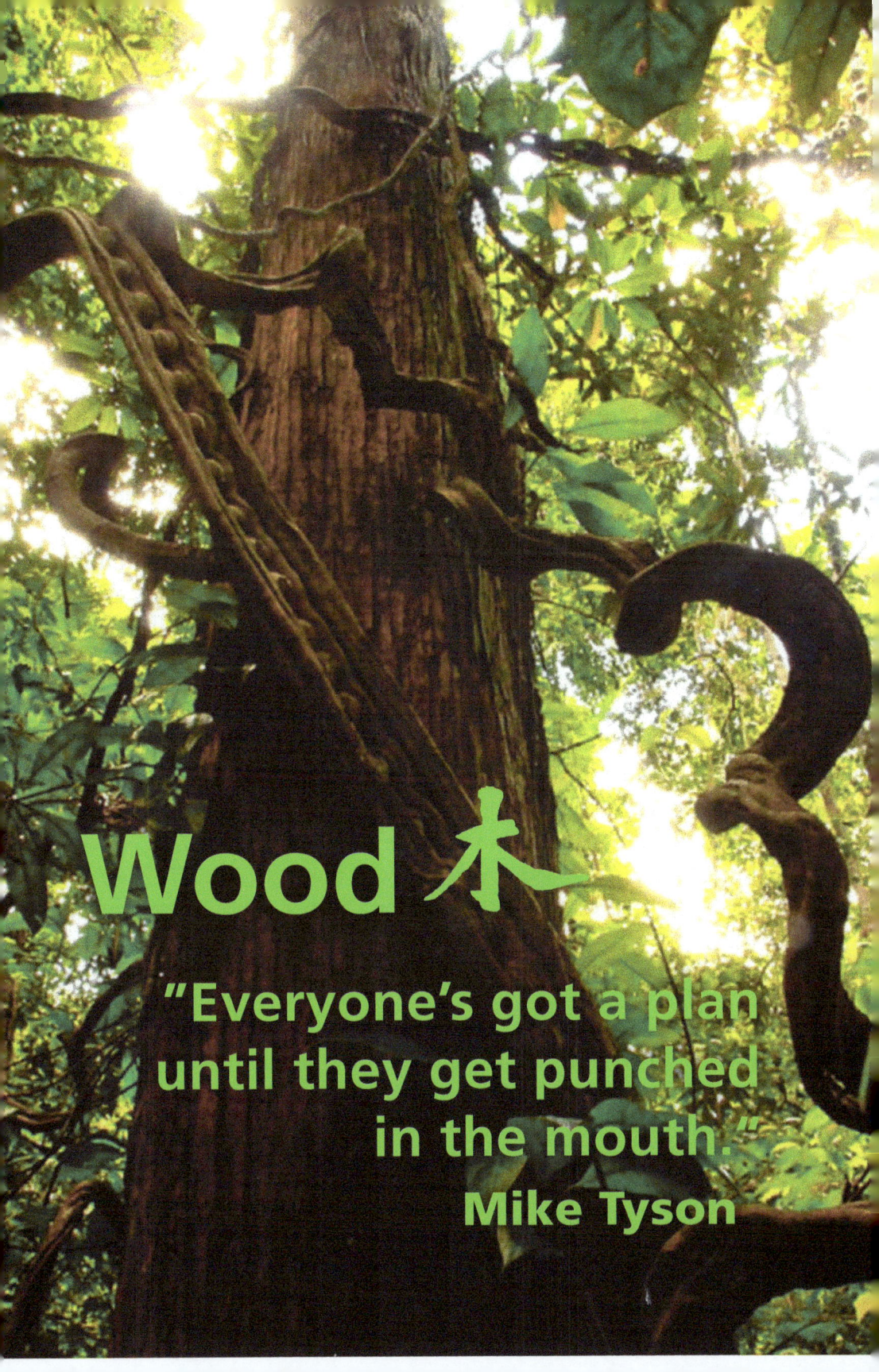

"Everyone's got a plan until they get punched in the mouth."
Mike Tyson

The Element Wood — Growth and Expansion

The strength of Wood manifests itself in the morning and in the East, in birth and in every new undertaking, in the freshness of the wind and in spring. In the Chinese tradition, the elements form a cycle which will be explained extensively in a later chapter. Wood is the first element of the cycle. It is called the young Yáng. In the body, Wood manifests itself in the Liver and Gallbladder, in the muscles and tendons, in the eyes and their tears. The Liver and Gallbladder produce the emotions which are ascribed to Wood: irritability, anger, fury, and rage. In the spirit, Wood brings forth the desire for movement and growth, it brings forth the creative process, planning and decision-making, and it gives us the desire to undertake a new project, to set sail for new horizons and new discoveries. The color associated with Wood is green.

The key to understanding this element is seen in the tree. The tree is rooted in the earth, often as deeply as its branches reach into the sky. Through its roots, the tree takes in water and minerals for its nourishment. It grows high into the sky, branches reaching out in all directions. For mankind, the tree has always symbolized growth in every direction, above and below, to the east and to the west, to the north and to the south. It has long been a symbol of expansive energy. In fall and in winter, it draws back into itself and gathers strength, for a new spring and summer, for a new growth ring.

Many ancient cultures worshiped trees. Many cultures considered the tree to be inhabited by spirits, for example, in China or in the Celtic culture. The Germans worshiped the oak. And the Essenes, a religious sect in ancient Palestine, portrayed the human being in the center of the tree of life: connected to energy lines as if in a magnetic field, the human stood in relation to the powers of heaven and earth. The figure was drawn in a meditative pose, the upper half of its body being the branches extending over the earth, and the lower half being the roots growing into the earth. The positions of the physical organs were also portrayed. The digestive, eliminative and reproductive organs in the lower half of the body represented the earthly component. The Lungs, Heart and Brain in the upper half of the body connected the person with the powers of the heavens. But the Liver and Gallbladder, the Wood organs, were portrayed at the center of the body, connecting what is above with what is below. This last example may show that cultures other than the Chinese saw the connection between the Liver and the tree.

The Liver is the Yin organ of the element Wood. Thus, it embodies the Yin energy of Wood: the ability to plan and see life on a material level as well as on an intellectual and spiritual level. The Liver embodies the power of imagination, the creative energy in us that results in growth. It is the inventor, the discoverer. It sees the meaning of life. It develops the vision, the plan. Every new idea that we take hold of, every new concept, broadens our horizons. We take risks and go into the unknown. We grow.

When the element Wood is healthy and balanced in a person, this human being is able to see that nature embodies an immense plan in which everything has its place and its role, and everything that happens, even the seemingly small and meaningless things, contributes to the pattern of events.

The cosmic plan goes beyond our power of imagination to such an extent that we can perceive the connection and inner meaning of a chain of events often only after a long time has passed. As long as we trust the cosmic plan, we keep a deep connection to the world. We grow with our environment, not against it.

The Yáng organ of Wood is the Gallbladder. It embodies the Yáng energy of this element: our ability to make decisions and to assert our needs in the outer world. One can compare the Liver to an architect who designs a house, while the Gallbladder is the builder who makes the decisions and arrangements that are necessary for the house to become a reality. The functions of both organs are closely connected to each other. Without an all-encompassing concept, the decisions in day-to-day life are incoherent, making little sense. At the same time, the best plans and projects are worthless if they cannot be carried out.

If planning and organization become a dry, bureaucratic routine, they will not lead to growth, but will often bring more harm than good. In the language of the Five Elements, inflexible and rigid planning is labeled "dry Wood" because it cracks and breaks under minimal pressure. Wood must be supple and full of sap for real growth to be possible.

In order to carry out a plan, we must take steps to realize it. We must "come out of ourselves" and fetch what we need to live. Therefore, it is understandable that the muscles and tendons are the bodily tissues assigned to Wood. If there is an obstacle to our growth — if we cannot find the space for expression — we feel frustrated and become angry. Anger and aggression are signs that our life energy is blocked, either from without or from within. In the theory of the Five Elements, anger and aggression are seen in a positive light: as emotions that help us to overcome impediments to our growth. Anger and aggression are the expression of a healthy Wood element, whereas irritability, hatred, rage, and fury are perceived as signs of an imbalance in Wood.

If rage is kept inside and cannot be cleared out, it seethes under a cold, numb, often polite surface. When it breaks out, it can become dangerous, as we all know. So it happens, again and again, that well-behaved, seemingly well-adjusted people commit murder or suicide in a fit of desperation.

Anger stands in contrast to rage. Anger is an energy that moves in the upper half of the body. It has more direction and focus than rage;

it can be more easily expressed. As mentioned above, anger helps us to clear obstacles out of our way so that we can carry through with our plans. In situations where the reason for being angry seems justified, one speaks of a "holy wrath." A well-known example of this is the scene in the Old Testament in which Moses comes down with the Ten Commandments from Mount Sinai and finds the Jews dancing around the golden calf, praying to an idol. As we know, he was overcome by a holy wrath that had important consequences for the further development of Judaism.

If there is an obstacle to our growth, if we cannot find the space for expression, we feel frustrated and become angry. Anger and aggression are a sign that our life energy is blocked either from without or from within. In the theory of the Five Elements, anger and aggression are seen in a rather positive light — as emotions that help us to overcome impediments to our growth. Anger and aggression are the expression of a healthy Wood element, whereas irritability, hatred, rage and fury are perceived as signs of an unbalance in Wood.

Rage and fury can be seen as undefined forms of aggression, with few possibilities for expression through language, gestures, or actions. Many people who have a constant rage lack the ability to recognize conflicts within themselves and express these to others. These people often did not learn in childhood to express their needs so as to receive what they wanted: their rage, or fury, built up over the years. Because they are often not capable of seeing their problems clearly, one also speaks of "blind rage." Rage is anger that has lost its purpose and gone out of control. Fury and rage typically lead to destructive behavior.

Annoyance and irritability also are emotions ascribed to the Wood element. They are also emotional energies that move in the upper half of the body but, in contrast to anger, they are very often symptoms of an emotional process in the unconscious where the energy has not yet been focused. In the language of the Five Elements, this is termed as "Wood which has not yet been gathered."

Anger as well as rage and fury are seen in Chinese medicine as an expression of the Wood Yáng. A choleric temperament, chronic irritability and unreasonable temper tantrums indicate a Shih state of the Gallbladder (a Gallbladder in the state of Fullness of Qì) which can also manifest itself as severe migraines in the temples or at the crown of the head. A longstanding Shih state of the Gallbladder — or a rage that cannot be clearly expressed, cleared out — often leads to high blood pressure or gallstones.

A lack of Yáng energy in Wood leads to suppressed rage, sarcasm, cynicism, bitterness, and, in general, an inability to get angry. It expresses itself in apathy, sluggishness, resignation, and depression. In these cases, there is too much Yin energy in Wood, either through an overactivity of Yin in the Liver or through a lack of Yáng in the Gallbladder.

The deep bitterness of people who have been gravely disappointed in life is the result of long years of frustration, usually stemming from being confronted constantly with obstacles to self-realization. It shows a long-standing imbalance in Wood. Irony, sarcasm, and cynicism are found in people who, often in their early childhood, lost the ability to easily approach and interact with other people. They are often the products of a strict intellectual or puritanical upbringing in which the expression of emotions and physical contact was taboo.

Apathy, resignation, and depression show that a person has given up making plans and manifesting goals. This outlook arises from continued failure; a person who is unable to act independently or to cany through with something eventually gives up. This often leads to alcoholism and addiction to drugs that are destructive to the Liver, as medication often is. In the Chinese tradition, the Liver is seen as the "House of Hún" or the "House of the Soul" — and the soul has become apathetic. Alcohol contributes to the maintenance of this condition, in which there is no room for new hopes that would question the acquired dismal view of the world.

Depression and resignation often have their roots in a disorder in Wood. The vision is missing, the plan is lacking (a lack of Qì in the Liver). Or a person might have many wishes and ideas, but just cannot put them into reality (a lack of Qì in the Gallbladder). As the Qì flows in the body from the Liver to the Lung Meridian, a lack of Qì in the Liver eventually leads to a depletion of Qì in the Lungs, causing shallow breathing, a sunken chest, and collapsed shoulders.

If, over the years, emotions such as hatred or rage cannot be expressed, cleared, and turned into a positive striving toward individual goals, the aggression often directs itself against one's own body. This can lead to illnesses such as gout, arthritis, rheumatism, and chronic poly arthritis — diseases in which the main symptoms are joint and muscle pains and an increasing restriction of movement.

So-called auto-immune diseases are also becoming more widespread and varied. In these illnesses, the body's cells produce antibodies that attack its own tissue. These are also appropriately called auto-aggressive diseases. The illnesses develop over years and decades; they are chronic and can be treated symptomatically by Western medical practices and eventually brought to a standstill, but they do not go away through medication. These diseases are found most often in women. In patriarchal cultures, women have less room than men to move and express themselves, especially when it comes to carrying through with an idea or venting anger.

To summarize, it is important for us to understand that, in the teachings of the Five Elements, anger and aggression are not put on the same level as destructive behavior, but rather understood as a basic impulse as the energy of Wood. The word "aggression" comes from the Latin verb *aggredi*, which means "to approach or tackle a thing or a person." If this normal expression of approaching someone or tackling something is hindered or restricted, it leads to a build-up of emotion; in the body, it leads to stiff muscles. This muscle tension is found, above all, in the neck, back, shoulders, and arms. Accumulated aggression is one of the major causes of headaches, neck pain, and back pain.

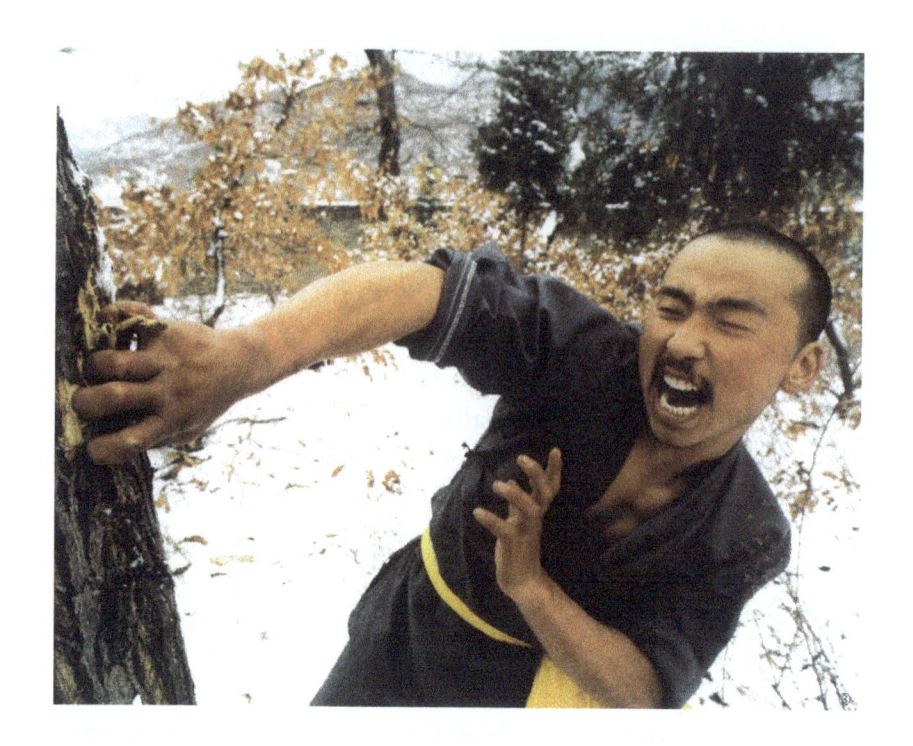

The growth of Wood occurs in all directions. If it has the necessary space and nourishment, then it grows balanced and symmetrical. Coordination and symmetry are essential characteristics of this element in nature, as well as in the lives of human beings. Most diseases in which symptoms occur only in one half of the body or those distinguished by a lack of coordination of the muscles, glands, and organs, can be traced to a disturbance in the element Wood.

Frequently, one can see an imbalance in Wood or can recognize it through an asymmetry in the face, or in the build of the body, or in a strong difference between the visual strength of the two eyes.

Because Wood governs the cycles of growth, when it is not balanced it causes disturbances such as growth disorders in childhood and puberty, irregular or painful menstruation, premature birth, or cancer. Other physical consequences of an imbalance in Wood are diseases of the eyes and problems with vision. These include near-sightedness and astigmatism (far-sightedness related to the aging process is more of a physiological development related to the tiring of the Wood element in later years). Other characteristic illnesses are high blood pressure and headaches behind the eyes, in the temples and at the crown of the head.

In the psychiatric and neurological area, an imbalance in Wood is exhibited in various mental illnesses, especially in schizophrenia and some forms of epilepsy. Schizophrenia is the crassest expression of a split personality — and an essential role of Wood is to bring mental, spiritual and physical components into equilibrium by coordinating the right and left hemispheres of the Brain. To a lesser degree, many people in our culture suffer from an impaired coordination of the left and right hemispheres of the Brain: this is reflected in the increasing number of people who need psychotherapy and heavy medication to keep their balance (and I'm talking here, for a change, about legal drugs). This comes from the development in recent decades that people have more and more difficulty in bringing thought, logic and rationality into harmony with intuition, fantasy, creativity and feelings because our educational system one-sidedly trains the left side of the Brain.

With epilepsy, the process is complex. Several elements contribute to the evolution of this disease. In most cases, epilepsy occurs because the relationship between Fire and Water is disturbed: if the Water element in a person has weakened, Water cannot put out the Fire (see the chapter on the Four Cycles at the end of the book) and, in certain stressful situations, the Fire blazes too high resulting in an epileptic fit which is nothing but a short circuit in the Brain.

The connection between epilepsy and the Wood element lies in the similarity between a major temper tantrum and an epileptic fit as well as in a deeper spiritual process which takes place during a fit and can perhaps only be completely understood by a shaman. I would like to point out that many seers and prophets, such as Moses, were epileptics or showed similar symptoms while in a trance. Many ancient cultures view epilepsy as a holy illness that allows the soul to enter into a dimension similar to that of the hereafter.

As emphasized by the enumeration of the diseases and disorders connected with Wood, this element is of great importance not only in diagnosis and therapy but also to better understand many diseases caused by civilization, such as migraine headaches, menstrual disorders, visual problems and high blood pressure. Above all, the increasingly common auto-aggressive diseases (in which the element Earth plays an important role along with Wood), are not completely understood by Western medical practitioners. They probably cannot be grasped in their entirety by a materially oriented culture because the causes lie mostly on mental and spiritual levels. Often these causes weaken an organ so much that infections or other illnesses can develop.

With disorders in Wood, the treatment can be difficult because Wood is the element of the hypochondriac. This makes sense if one considers that confusion and disorder reign when plans and decisions are lacking. In such cases, symptoms come and go, or they seem to wander naturally from one part of the body to another. A weak constitution and symptoms that always appear in spring also indicate a Wood-related illness, as spring is the time when Wood releases its strength.

When Wood is balanced, springtime brings new interests and goals along with ambition and vitality. In contrast, when Wood is sick, spring will be a time of frustration, bringing tiredness and depression. Statistics show that the suicide rate rises in the spring. With a traditional treatment according to the teachings of the Five Elements, it is possible to restore balance so that new growth can be promoted. Then the vital energy that spring brings to Wood can carry through into the warmth of summer, the ripening period of late summer, the harvest time of fall, and the restful period of winter, when seeds can begin to germinate in preparation for a new cycle of growth.

Just as it is possible to see the workings of the Five Elements on a person's physical, mental, and spiritual levels, one can also see their influence in interpersonal relations in different cultural and social structures. Cultural, national, and social systems create structures analogous to the human organism. Several ancient civilizations see our earth as an enormous organism, with humankind as the central nervous system. This analogy makes it clear how easily the breakdown of a part of this gigantic central nervous system jeopardizes the well-being of the total organism.

In Europe, North America, and Japan, the worst consequences of an imbalance in Wood can be observed. In these highly industrialized countries, a schism exists in the relationship with this Element. In the language of the Elements, the division can be described as a very strong, self-conscious Wood-Yáng that is pitted against a weak, undernourished, confused Wood-Yin.

On the one hand, these countries have been expanding magnificently for a long time. They have made technological advances, built strong military forces, and spread their religions. They have imposed their wills and their worldviews onto many other people. Many inventions and discoveries have arisen out of these cultures. On the other hand, it is striking to witness the meaninglessness and growing insecurity that plague many people in the large, developed cities of these "advanced" regions. And there is a deep-seated confusion and lack of direction in connection with the global discussion of ecology, the dying out of the forests, and the debate about nuclear weapons.

There is a lot of discussion and a lot of information, but no vision. These discussions deliver many messages, but without much mature contemplation. The ability to have visions and to recognize how things are connected is no longer respected, and because of this, it is not developed. Visionaries are handled with mistrust; Socrates and Christ were poisoned and crucified. Others were slandered, not understood, put in prison, silenced, or executed. There are numerous examples: witches and magicians in the Middle Ages, Paracelsus, Franz Anton Mesmer, Georg Büchner, Friedrich Nietzsche, Sigmund Freud, Wilhelm Reich, Mahatma Gandhi, and Martin Luther King Jr., to name a few. In other cultures, a certain amount of unusual behavior from seers and prophets was endured or even encouraged. They were given the right to criticize and inform the ruling party; this was permitted of court fools in the Middle Ages. On the contrary, in our culture, wise men and fools are ridiculed.

Vision is the power of Wood. Usually, before a new vision can take shape, confusion, dissolution and chaos rule. In other cultures, therefore, the elders both tolerated the temperament of the fools and respected their wisdom. A further crossroads in our relationship with Wood manifests itself in our attitude toward aggression. On the one hand, aggression is described in Christian teaching as being bad and wicked. In interpersonal relationships, a loud word or a strong gesture is frequently judged negatively. The natural expression of playful aggression was often restricted and suppressed in childhood.

On the other hand, Western culture is one of the most aggressive cultures that has ever existed. It has "made the world its subject," as the Bible puts it. The extent of the destruction that has been inflicted by this culture does not need to be described here. The curbing and suppression of aggression in interpersonal relationships has led to an enormous build-up of rage that discharges itself again and again on a cultural and national level. So we find ourselves in a paradoxical situation, in which the leaders of the industrialized world speak about peace and safety, and instead give birth to destruction. They bring advancement and progress to other cultures, thus destroying them. Most scientific theories of aggression tend not to account for the effect of aggression on a national and cultural level.

Aggression is our "blind spot." How else could it be explained that there are still scientific symposiums and publications? It is judged by orthodox psychology as pathological and destructive, as something that should be treated and transformed.

Another current opinion in Western culture is that anger and aggression should be sublimated and transformed into love and peace. This would be ideal, but it only works if the anger has been properly expressed and has turned naturally to joy and love. We can watch this phenomenon with small children who, after a brisk and rough fight, become easily reconciled with each other. If the anger is suppressed and not expressed, and people try to be kind and polite under all circumstances, real feelings are replaced by unnatural behavior patterns. This often results in a false spirituality, in which creativity and spontaneity are subtly cut off and slowly vanish from the personality.

A further cause of the negativity projected onto aggression lies in its close association with sexuality. As observed in the investigations of anthropologists and researchers such as Margaret Mead and Wilhelm Reich, inhibited and suppressed aggression goes hand in hand with inhibited and suppressed sexuality. Stated in positive terms, healthy aggressive behavior is a condition of healthy sexual behavior, and healthy sexual behavior is related to healthy aggressive behavior. This connection is also portrayed in Chinese paintings.

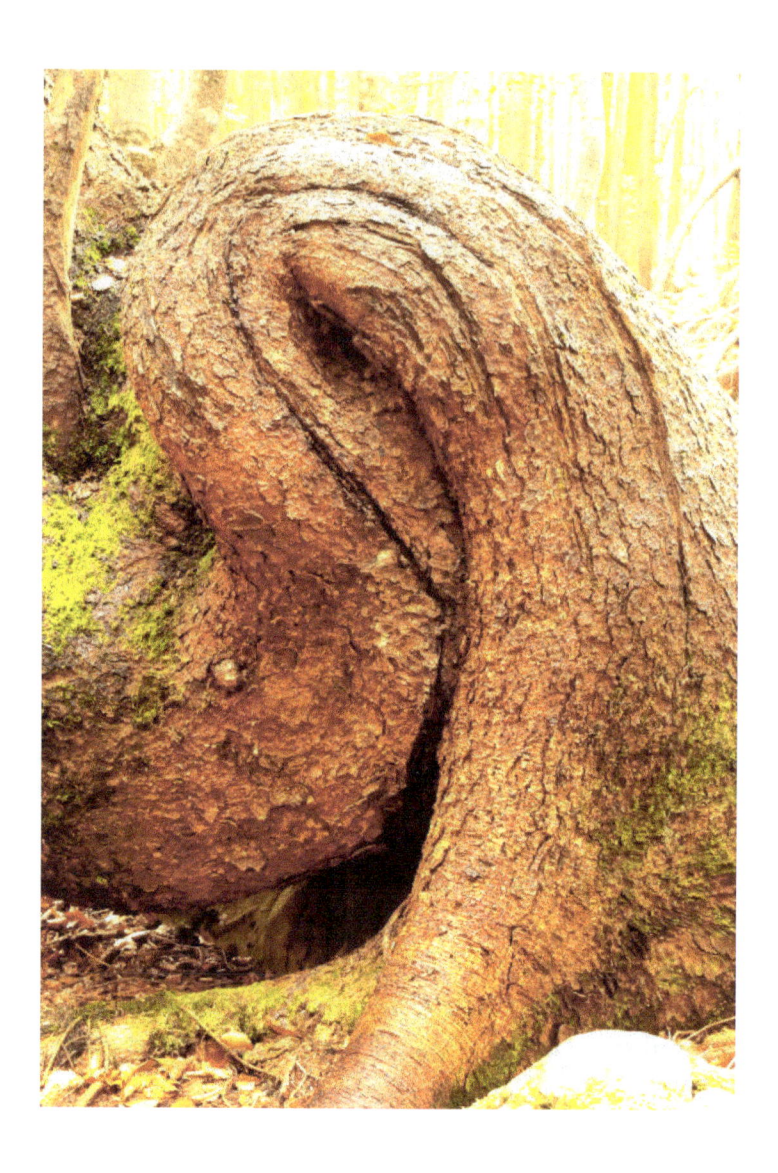

Wood naturally expands, flowing gently, continuously, and unimpeded. If you love someone physically, spiritually, or intellectually, you extend yourself into that person's space. When you hug another person, the space you are in expands. This simple phenomenon of gentle expansion and connecting with another — creating a larger space than the separate self — is love, which belongs to the element Wood.

The problems that Western culture has with Wood show themselves here also. On the one hand, love is highly prized and mystified, yet on the other hand, it is restricted and detached from the physical. Conditions are placed on the avenues of its expression and it is clothed in strict rituals. The flower children of the sixties were pursued and discriminated against by the police. "Make love not war!" stood for an anticultural, immoral provocation.

Interestingly, the term "love" rarely shows up in old Chinese texts. In *I Ching (The Book of Changes),* there is no hexagram that represents our idea of love. There is Peace, The Receptive, The Creative, The Aroused, The Gentle, The Serene, and The Obliging, but our concept of love does not appear. Only in the newer commentaries on *I Ching* does one find this term.

In an ancient Chinese text called *Da Dsuan, The Large Discourse,* it is written as follows:

> In that the person becomes like the heavens and the earth, he does not come to be opposed to them. His wisdom embraces all things and his mind orders the whole world. Because of this, he does not make any mistakes. He has an effect on everything, but he does not let himself be carried away by anything. He is joyful of the heavens and knows fate. Thus, he is free of worries. He is satisfied with his situation and sincere in his goodness. Therefore, he is capable of expressing love.

Mental and Physical Exercises to Stimulate the Growth of Wood

While reading this section, you have probably already noticed some information that is relevant to your own life. Perhaps you have also asked yourself how this knowledge can influence your health, your feelings, or your worldview.

It makes a big difference whether you read about the art of running and its positive effects and then find the time and energy to run, or if you allow the theory to be enough. In order to go beyond an intellectual understanding of the elements, I have put together some exercises to give you direct experience with each element. With these, you can touch, hear, smell, taste, and see things that the printed word cannot convey. These experiences take place in your body and become anchored in your senses and movements; they become integrated into your self.

Clarifying questions

The questions in this chapter have to do with your Wood element. You will find out in which areas you depart from the description of "healthy Wood."

Give yourself at least half an hour without interruptions to calmly and reflectively answer all of the following questions. Make yourself comfortable. Read a question, then close your eyes and let the question sink into you. Our waking consciousness is often ready to give quick answers that are only partially true. Pay attention to the first answer that comes into your head and to paradoxical answers that do not seem to fit into the picture.

Life is a state of maintaining relative balance between various states of constantly changing imbalances. Small deviations from the norm are typical of a lively life. In all areas of our existence, we sway back and forth between two poles. If we remain stuck on the Yin or Yáng pole for any length of time and we do not express the other pole, our growth and maturation will be restricted and our physical and mental health will be harmed. Examples of opposite poles are: waking vs. sleeping, relaxed vs. active or tense, anger vs. gentleness.

Use the following questions to get to know the condition of your Wood element and to discover any imbalances you may have. For example, there is something wrong with your Wood element if you are always irritable and explode at the slightest provocation, but there is also something wrong if you are unable to get angry at all in a situation where people seriously mistreat you. Some other examples are as follows: there is something wrong with your Wood if you have major vision problems; if you cannot stand sour taste, or if you have a deep craving for sour food; or if you easily get irritable and hysterical in windy weather.

These questions cannot simply be answered by yes or no, and nobody is there to tell you how many points you have scored in the Wood element. Use these questions to develop a sense of whether your Wood element is more or less balanced. If you get the impression that your Wood element is either too strong or too weak, do the subsequent exercises that can help you win back your balance. Do the mental and emotional exercises such as "Vision of the future" and "Unexpressed anger" a few times within a month, and do the exercises to stimulate the flow of Qì in the Liver and Gallbladder Meridians on a daily basis for three weeks if you want some change.

- How do I feel in the morning?
- How do I feel in spring?
- How do I feel on windy days?

- Do I have a special craving for/a strong aversion to acidic (sour) food or drink?
- Are my Liver and Gallbladder healthy, or have I had jaundice, gallstones or a bilious attack?
- Are my muscles strong or weak?
- Do I enjoy movement?
- Am I physically active?
- Do I have a tendency toward inflamed tendons or pulled muscles?
- Do I sometimes 'freeze up' in situations, but do not let anyone see it and become angry after the fact?
- How do I express anger and frustration?
- How often do I swallow my anger instead of losing my temper?
- Do I have a tendency towards irony or cynicism?
- Is there anything in my personal history that makes me feel bitter?
- Do I frequently feel a thirst for revenge?
- Is there anyone I really hate?
- Am I often irritable or moody?
- Can I attain my goals and carry through with my intentions most of the time?
- Do I have an image of how I would like to live, and does my reality correspond to this image?
- How good is my eyesight?
- How do I approach new situations?

Wood exercises

Vision of the future

Spend an evening alone. Take a bath and put on light, comfortable clothes. Seek a quiet place where you can relax undisturbed.

Lie on your back, close your eyes, and breathe deeply and regularly for about a minute, like a sleeping child. Then imagine that you are journeying into the picture of your life that you carry within you. Paint the details of how you would like to live. Dream yourself into a world where there are no restrictions or limitations. If a good fairy could help you to realize your wishes, what occupation would you like to have? With which partner would you live? How much time would you have for yourself and your personal interests? How would your relationships with other people be?

Do not let yourself be disturbed at this time by negative or critical thoughts. Ignore the doubter, the one who is resigned and cynical. Every thought can become a reality, but you have to give it time to take root and develop.

The best time for a future vision is in February or March, but you can do this exercise at other times, especially before making important decisions. A vision gains strength when you write it down in a journal and when you visualize it often in vivid detail.

Unexpressed anger

If you have difficulty venting your anger in the presence of other people, try the following exercise.

Withdraw to a room or look for a place in the open air where you will not be disturbed. Imagine a concrete situation in which you did not dare to let your anger run free. See the person with whom you were in conflict symbolically in a pillow. Spontaneously express your opinion as if the person were standing directly in front of you. Allow yourself to become powerful, to raise your voice, shout, rant, and become physical. Exaggerate a bit and let yourself go in the situation.

Everyday irritation

Practice expressing aggressive behavior for a few days. Invite situations that arouse your anger and seek out meetings with people who you know will drive you up the wall. Express your anger energetically. Observe yourself when you are angry. Observe the reactions of others. Is it how you thought it would be?

I know this is a tough one. The purpose of the exercise is to de-automatize the way you deal with difficulties and hindrances. If you have a difficult time getting angry at all, this exercise should prove to be particularly helpful: You "exercise" an assertive response to have it on hand when you really need it. Because in the actual situation where there is a major difficulty, there are always multiple reasons to not speak up.

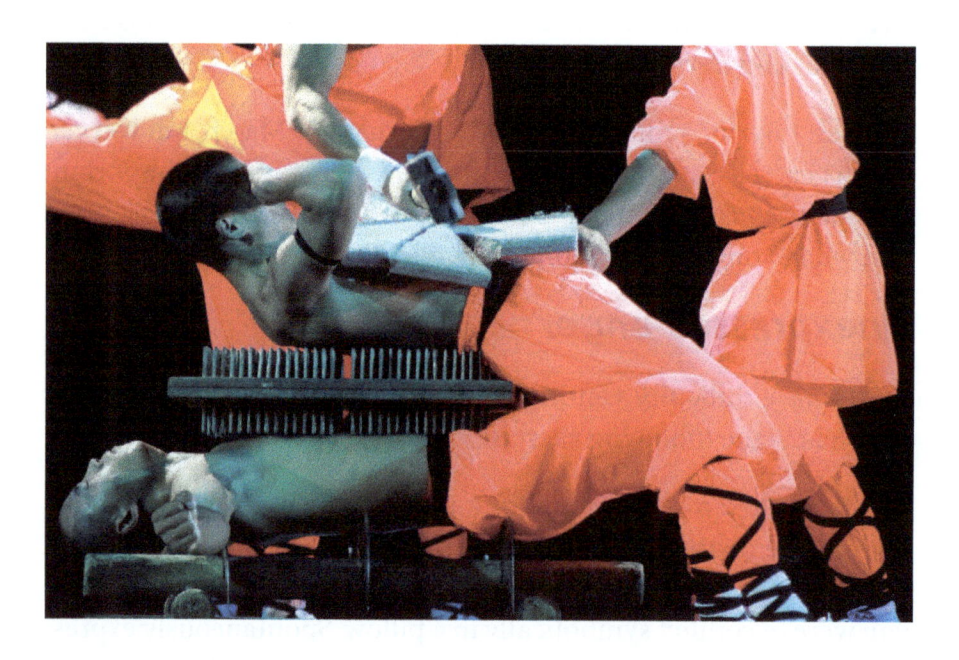

If you are a hothead, this exercise is helpful in order to become conscious of your anger patterns. If you deliberately set up a situation in which to become angry, you are beginning to master your aggression and your anger pattern will change because awareness transforms the automatic emotional response.

Movement

Physical movement that causes perspiration strengthens the element Wood. Along with heavy physical work, most sports fulfill this purpose. Martial arts (for example Judo, Karate, and Aikido) especially strengthen a weak Wood element and combat excess body weight.

Exercises for the Gallbladder and Liver Meridians

You know how it is with exercises. We would rather think about them than do them. But if you want to strengthen an element, you need to do the meridian exercises of the corresponding element on a daily basis for a minimum of three weeks. After the three weeks, evaluate the effect these exercises are having on your body and on your mental and emotional life. Then decide whether to do the exercises daily for three months. If you do the following exercises on a regular basis, you will increasingly experience the strength of Wood in your body and in your actions; you will feel fitter and more decisive, and your vision will probably improve.

For each organ, two exercises are described. They strengthen the flow of Qì through the organ and its corresponding meridian. Thus, they enhance the physiological, emotional, mental, and spiritual functions of the organ. The first exercise consists of a physical posture combined with a visualization of the corresponding meridian. This exercise also helps you to develop a feeling for the quality of the corresponding organ and element. The second exercise directly activates the flow of Qì in the actual meridian.

Strengthening the Wood-Yáng

The Gallbladder posture

The posture shown in the photograph depicts the essence of the Chinese understanding of the Gallbladder. It represents the spirit of beginning, setting out on something new, making a decision, and being driven. It depicts life as "the way," and the significance of traveling actively along that path.

This posture will introduce you to the flow of the Gallbladder Meridian. Imagine a red or orange stream of energy about two inches wide that begins at your right eye and flows downward to your feet; this is the meridian. Strengthen the image in your imagination every time you exhale.

Then begin to walk slowly back and forth, continuing to concentrate on the flow of the meridian. After two or three minutes, repeat the exercise visualizing the Gallbladder Meridian on your left side.

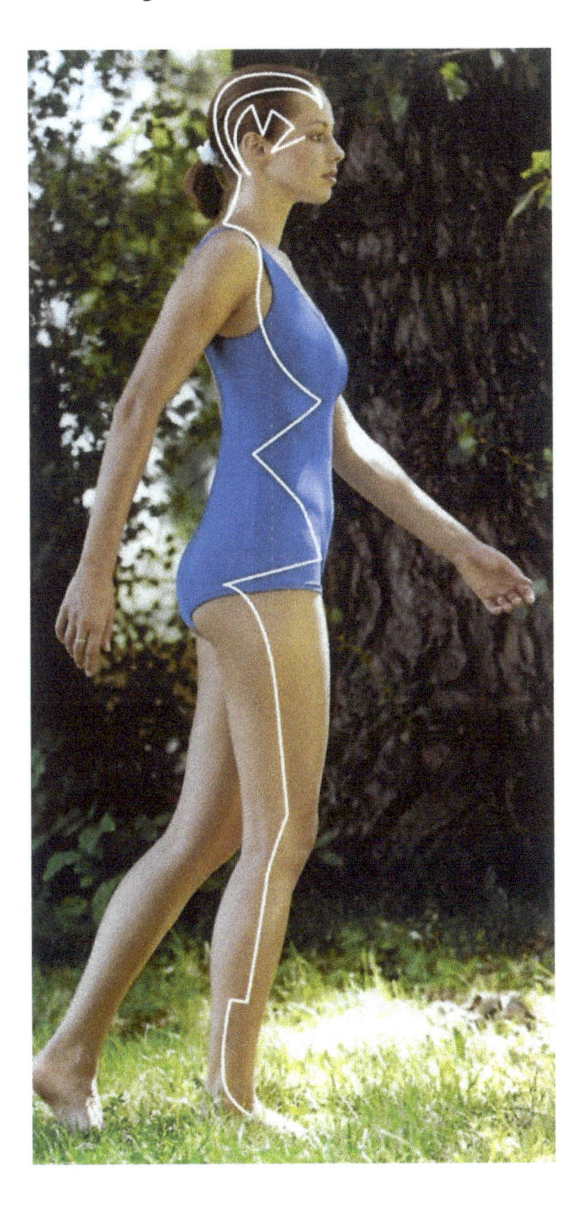

Activating the Gallbladder Meridian

1. Stand with your feet parallel, spread a couple of feet apart. Your shoulders should be relaxed, arms hanging loosely at your sides. Your knees should be slightly bent.

2. Extend your arms straight above your head, with the palms of your hands facing each other.

3. Inhaling, bend your body as far to the left as you can. Your arms should remain as straight as possible. As you stretch to the side, keep your torso aligned and look straight ahead. Let the weight of your right arm stretch your right side so that you have the feeling of a taught bow extending down into your right foot.

4. Stand up straight again. Exhale intensely and, with your hands made into fists, move in one sudden movement into a stooped position with your knees slightly bent.

5. As you inhale, stand up straight and repeat the exercise, this time bending to the right.

6. Repeat this exercise 10 times on each side.

Wood • 39

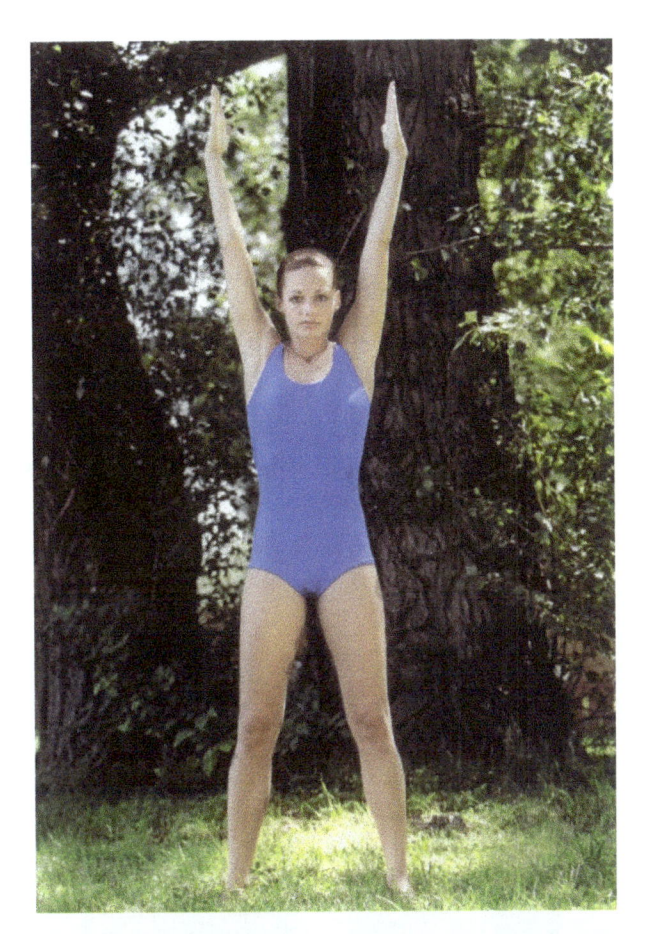

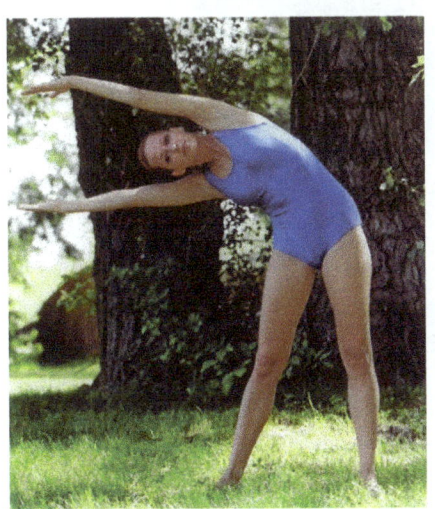

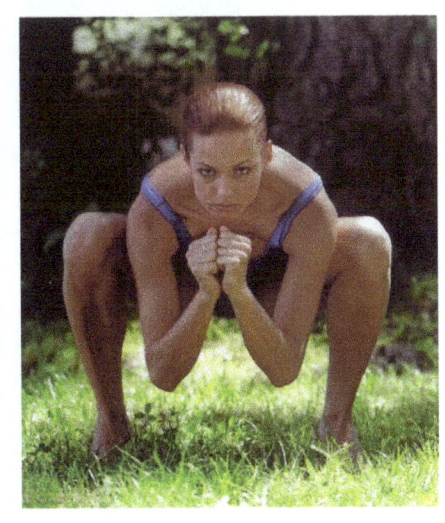

Strengthening the Wood-Yin

The Liver posture

This posture embodies the essence of the Liver energy: the tree, physical growth, balance, coordinated strength, and quiet concentration on the essential.

Visualize your Liver Meridian as a river of energy that flows from your big toe up to your chest. Strengthen your visualization of this flow with every inhalation. Stay in this posture for at least a minute. Then repeat the exercise with the other leg. If you have difficulty maintaining your balance, it is a sign that you are not rooted enough in yourself.

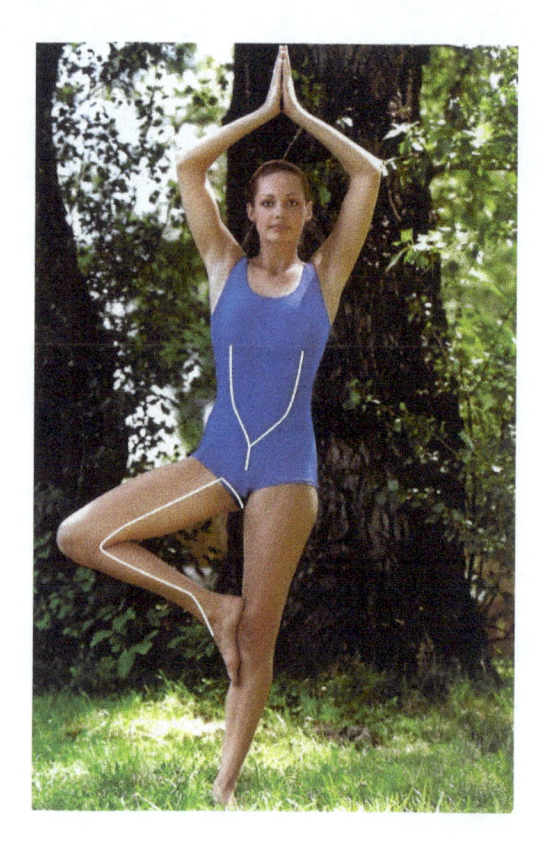

Activating the Liver Meridian

1. Lie on your back and bring your ankles toward your buttocks so that your knees are bent and pointing to the ceiling. Hold your ankles with your hands. Your feet should be flat on the floor.

2. Breathe in while raising your hips as high as possible from the ground, and breathe out while lowering your body back to the floor.

3. Repeat this exercise for a minute. Then lift your hips one last time as high as possible and remain in this position. At the same time, tighten your buttocks and stomach muscles as much as possible. Then let yourself sink back into a state of relaxation.

4. Lie flat on your back with your eyes closed and be aware of your body.

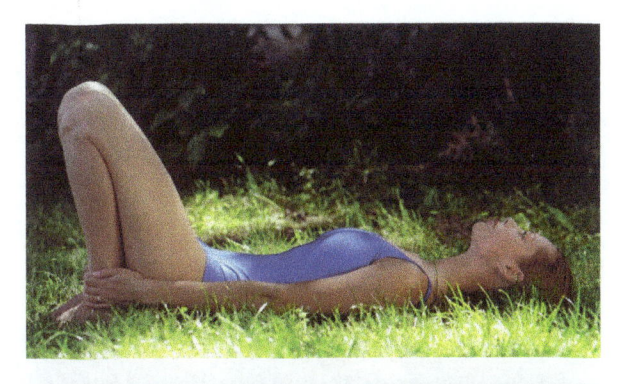

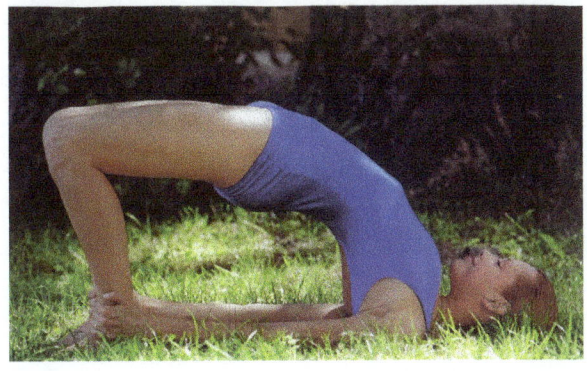

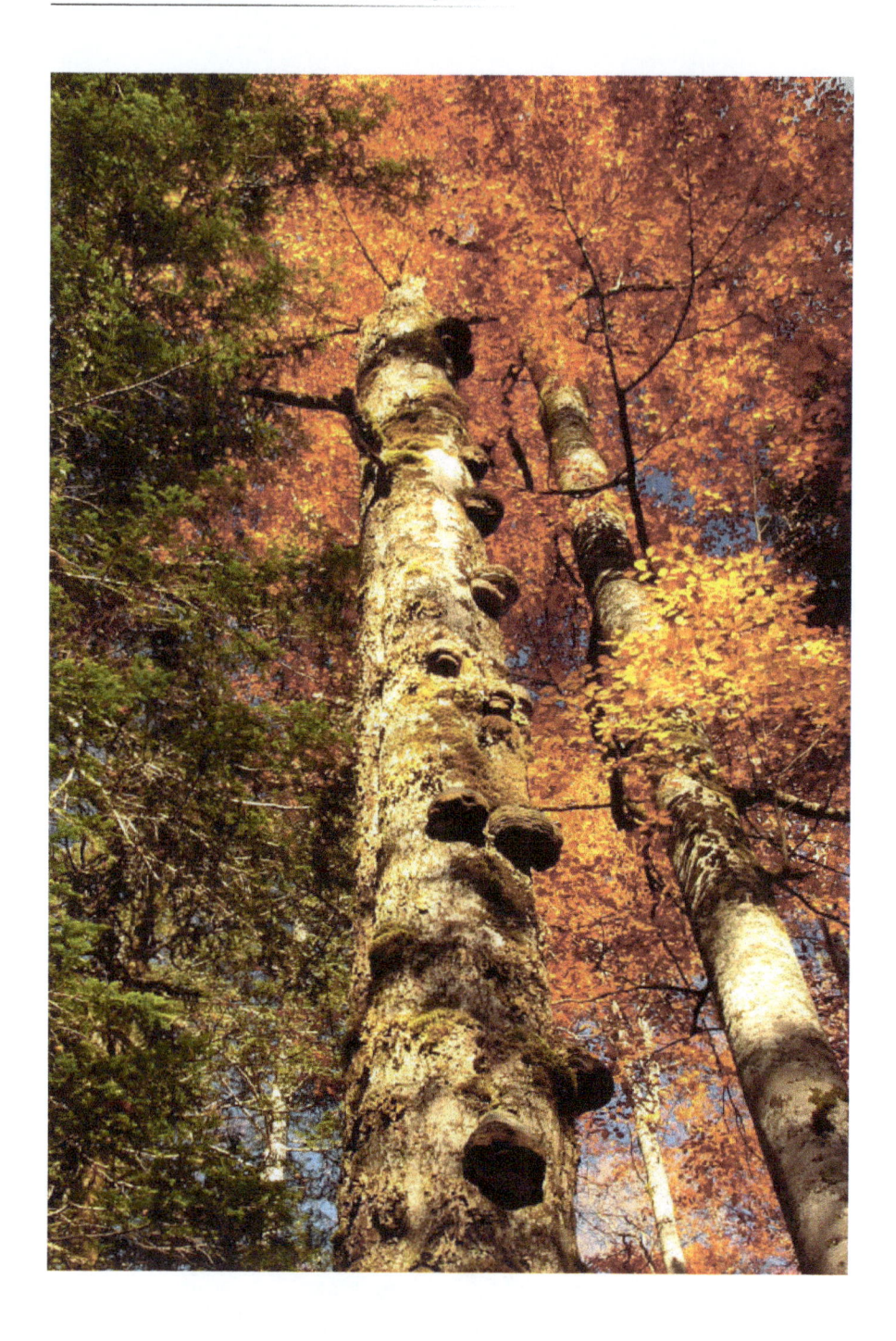

Fire 火

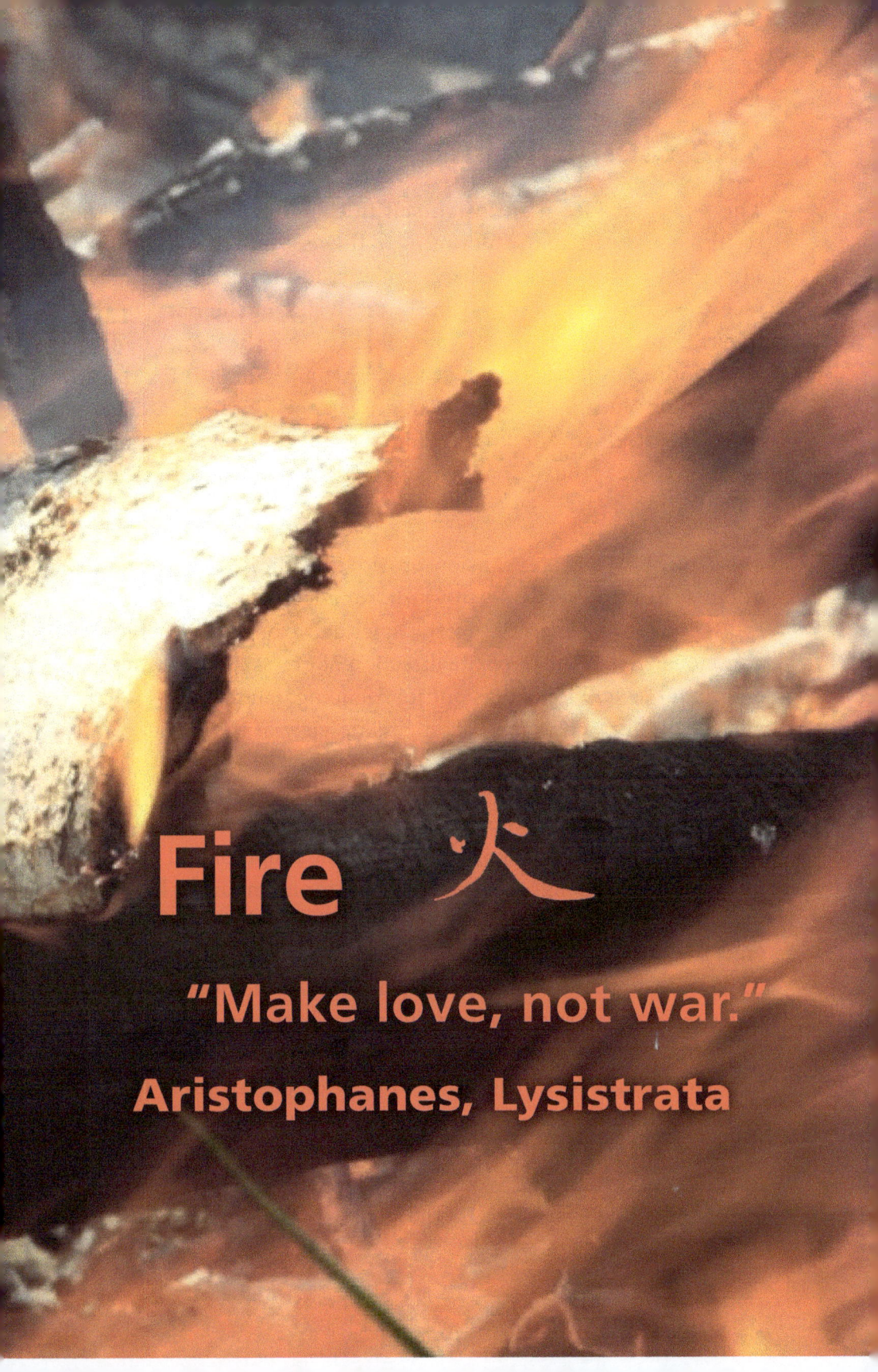

"Make love, not war."
Aristophanes, Lysistrata

The Element Fire

The power of Fire manifests itself in the afternoon and in the south, in warmth, in the blooming of flowers, and in the summer. Fire follows Wood in the Shéng cycle: Wood is used to make fire (see the chapter regarding the Four Cycles in the back of this book). Fire is called the old Yáng. Fire is the only element which is embodied in four organs: in the Heart and Small Intestine, in the Pericardium or Heart Cover, and in the Triple Heater. Fire manifests itself in our tongue and speech. It governs the blood vessels: the capillaries, arteries, and veins. Its bodily fluid is perspiration.

The nature of Wood is expansion, growth in all directions. The power of Fire is directed vertically upward, from deep in the earth up into the sky, from the material to the spiritual, from unawareness to consciousness, in the opposite direction of gravity. On the mental-emotional level, Fire brings out joy, dancing, laughter, awareness, and the ability to have an encompassing view of things. Its colors are scarlet and red.

Ancient China had a court culture with a strict hierarchy. The social order, which was centered around the Emperor and his royal household, was thought to be responsible for maintaining harmony between heaven and earth. In contrast to Greek philosophy (which emerges from the cosmos and the laws of nature) and the Indian philosophy of the Vedas and the Upanishads (which recognizes the inner self as the essence of the universe), Chinese cosmology finds its central themes in the order of society and ethics: Correct personal behavior brings forth the proper behavior of nature. If society, especially the Emperor and his court members in the center, followed the laws of the Tao, then the land would be spared hardships, including floods, droughts, epidemics, hunger, and typhoons. This social-mystical viewpoint held the society together.

This belief also permeated Chinese medicine in that the human body was seen as the court, and the different organs as the civil servants. If individuals fulfilled their social responsibilities, honored their ancestors, placated their demons, and maintained contact with the Elements operating through their organs, thoughts, and actions, then illnesses stayed away from them.

The first Yin organ of Fire is the Heart. It is called the Fire Prince, the highest ruler of the organs. It is seen as the center of consciousness, feelings, and thoughts. Yin Shén, the spirit of Fire, rules the Heart. The Chinese character Shén can be translated as "spirit," "soul," "God," "godly," and "effectiveness." The meaning of this character is touched upon when one says that a person has spirit.

Shén has two houses. The lower residence is the Heart, where it ensures balanced feelings and a clear, honest way of speaking. Its higher house is the third eye, or forehead chakra (a Hindu term for energy center), where it brings forth clarity of thoughts and a conscious life direction. When these characteristics are present in a person, that person's Shén is powerful and healthy. One recognizes this as a sparkle or light in the eyes.

If, however, Shén is confused or lacking in energy, it is noticeable in unclear thinking or an inability to organize thoughts, in speech defects ranging from lisping, stammering, or stuttering to muteness, or in emotions full of highs and lows, one minute shouting for joy, the next minute wanting to die. This includes different forms of hysteria and manic depression. A dispersed, confused Shén expresses itself in nervousness, fearfulness, stage fright, insomnia, and dull, unfocused eyes. All of these symptoms are caused by a disturbance in the Fire element.

When the Fire energy in the Heart is too strong, the Chinese say it is Shí, in excess. This results in talkativeness, excessive perspiration, and nervous tension. People with this condition believe that they have to take everything into their own hands; they must control everything. Most of the time they are not capable of letting other people take responsibility. This is a characteristic of contemporary "manager sickness," which often leads to heart failure. The "Type A" personality and its stress-related illnesses, characterized by high blood pressure and heart attacks, are manifestations of Shí in the Heart. As we see later, this imbalance typically emerges as a result of an energy deficit in the Water element.

When the Fire energy in the Heart is too weak, it is called Xu, deficient. This leads to disturbances, such as inability to express oneself clearly, partial or total muteness, and a dulled or nonfunctioning sense of taste, both on the tongue and in the psyche.

The second Yin organ of Fire is the Pericardium, also called the Heart Cover or Heart Governor. It is designated in the Chinese tradition as the first minister or chancellor of the Fire Prince, as bodyguard and protector of the Heart, and as its castle. Its task is to protect the prince from harm and defeat, to give orders to the court officials and subjects, and to report to the prince about his well-being. In people, it brings about the ability to be generous to oneself and to others, to radiate warmth, and to love. The Heart Governor expresses itself in the ability to give and in the ability to accept complaints, lamentations, criticism, and love from others. When this characteristic is developed, a person is able to speak from the Heart and be cordial and affectionate, enthusiastic, humorous, and hearty. In contrast, we speak of some people as being cold-hearted or small-minded, as if they have a heart of stone. A serious form of inflammation of the Pericardium can lead to a so-called "armored heart" on an organic level.

In Chinese physiology, the duties of the Heart and the Pericardium also include the maintenance and regulation of the circulatory system. Accordingly, the arteries and veins are categorized as the "tissue" of Fire. The Heart, Pericardium, blood vessels, and all the hormones and regulatory mechanisms having to do with the maintenance and control of the circulatory system through dilation or contraction of the blood vessels form a functional unit.

In ancient Chinese texts, the Pericardium is spoken of as the Yáng-Kidney. In modern Chinese medicine, the term "Yáng-Kidney" refers to the suprarenal glands, whose main function, besides regulating the metabolism, is to control the circulatory system and the fluid and electrolyte levels. This means that, in ancient times, the Pericardium was thought of as pertaining to the Water element, whereas, in this century, the Pericardium is considered the second Fire Yin organ. But it is important to remember that the functions of the Yáng-Kidney and the Pericardium are closely linked together and that the Pericardium occupies a central position between the Kidney and the Heart, between Water and Fire, between the upper and lower poles of a person.

To further understand this, it should be noted that the Chinese recognize six different energy layers in the human organism, each layer being nourished, maintained, and regulated by two organs. The innermost layer, the core of our body and personality, is made up of the Kidney and the Heart. These two organs build our vertical axis, our basic polarity of Hara and head. Heart and Kidney form the polarity of Fire and Water, of above and below, of Heaven and Earth, of God and the Devil, of Zeus and Hades, and of Jupiter and Pluto.

In India, the worship of Shiva, the destroyer, is placed on the same level as those of Brahma, the creator, and Vishnu, the maintainer. In China, the balance between above and below, and right and left, is seen as desirable. However, in Western civilization, a higher value is placed on the upper pole. This belief has led to a one-sided effort — a striving that is directed "above," to the "good," "to get into heaven" — and with that, to the creation of evil and our concept of hell. In Western cultures, the areas of Fire — love, speech, and intellect — are more treasured than the depths of Water — sexuality, meditation, and sinking into the archaic levels of the soul. Just think of the beginning of the Gospel according to John: "In the beginning was the word, and the word was with God, and God was the word. And the word became flesh and dwelled among us."

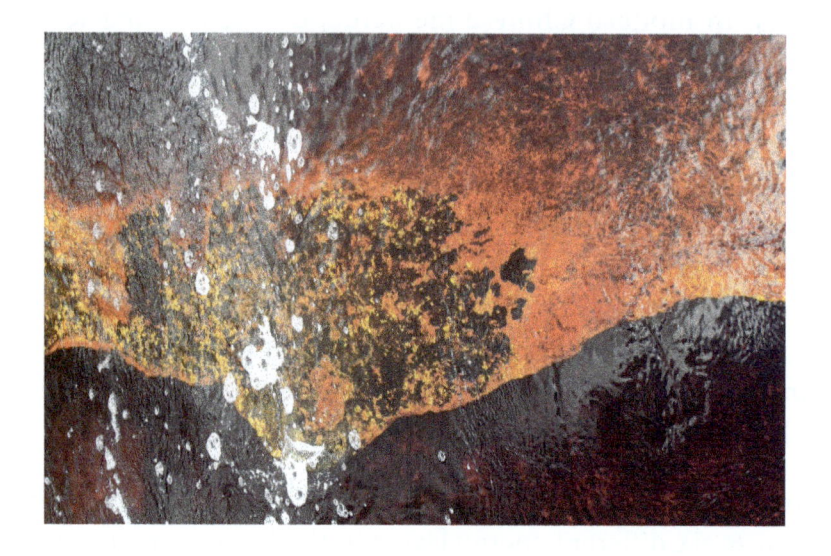

If the Pericardium is in balance, it forms a bridge between Water and Fire and we experience a fulfilled sexuality which brings forth joy and laughter. If the Qì flows in the Pericardium, we feel a deep connection between sexual lust and love, and we are able to freely give and receive. In this context, it might be interesting to note that, in the Seventies, in its attempt to free sexuality from damnation, our culture had to pay much more attention to the physical orgasm, which is a function of the Water element, than to the needs of the soul. Only in the Eighties also due to the advent of Aids did the union of Water and Fire in love and sexuality become more important again.

Although the Heart and Pericardium are two Yin organs belonging to the same element, they have vastly different tasks. The Heart is responsible for "inner matters." Its functions include clarity of thought, speech, responsibility, and motivation. This is also expressed in the names of a few of the points on the Heart Meridian. Shén Mén (Heart 7) means "Gate of the Spirit" or "Gate of the Consciousness." Tong Li (Heart 5) means "Relationship to the Inner." On the other hand, the Pericardium is responsible for "outer matters," regulating blood circulation, heartbeat, and heart frequency on the organic level. Cold hands and feet are a symptom of a lack of energy in the Pericardium. A person with little warmth has an energy deficit in the Pericardium. This includes people who do not find much joy in sexuality, stingy people who have a difficult time giving, people who need a long time to thaw, and closed people who don't laugh.

Due to this, points on the Heart Meridian are usually used in treating psychological disorders, for example, insomnia, nervousness, hysteria, manic depression, and epilepsy. They are also used to treat speech disorders and people who have difficulty listening to others. However, the points on the Pericardium Meridian are more likely to help when there is a physical problem with the Heart, for example, heart pains, angina pectoris, tachycardia, heartbeat irregularities, or circulatory problems. But, of course, points on the Pericardium channel also have a marked psychological effect.

The Small Intestine is the Yáng organ assigned to the Heart. The key to understanding its function is seen in the assimilation of nourishment in the digestive process. Just as the Small Intestine takes care that nourishment can be absorbed in the blood, it is also responsible on an intellectual level for the assimilation of ideas. An energy deficit in the Small Intestine is manifested in a person who takes on knowledge, convictions, and beliefs from others undigested and is not capable of developing personal views and belief systems out of this. The appearance of a person who is able to assimilate is displayed through a fine, silent laughing in the eyes and around the lips.

The Triple Heater, or San Jiao, is the second Yáng organ of Fire, being assigned to the Pericardium. The Triple Heater is an association of various functions in the body and mind, rather than an organic reality.

The Chinese teachings speak of the San Jiao as the "three burning cavities" in the organism: the chest (for breathing), the abdomen (for digestion), and the pelvis (for excretion and reproduction). The task of the Triple Warmer is to coordinate these three areas of the body, for instance, coordinating the depth and frequency of breath in relation to digestion and sexuality, and regulating body temperature and equilibrium. It is assumed that the Chinese term San Jiao also includes the different centers for the regulation of body temperature in the Brain, especially the hypothalamus.

The Triple Warmer is the most complex of the organs, and because of this, it is also the easiest to bring out of balance in the entire organism. In classical texts, it appears as the foreign minister of Fire, the protector of the Yin and Yáng organs, the energy minister who oversees the production of the different types of Qì and guarantees its distribution in the body.

When the Fire element in a person is balanced, summer brings joy and fulfillment. Such people have an inner balance out of which they engage with events. They know when to speak and when to remain silent. They can feel joy without becoming excessive. They can steer and lead others, but they know when the time is right to pull back. Their eyes glow. They know goodness and magnanimity, and they have good taste.

Mental and Physical Exercises to Ignite the Fire

Clarifying questions

Proceed with the following questions as you have done with Wood:

- How do I feel in summer, in the heat, or in the south?
- Do I perspire easily?
- Do I talk too much or too little?
- Can I satisfyingly communicate my needs and ideas?
- Can I react spontaneously to an unforeseen and unexpected situation?
- Do I listen attentively to others, or do I think about what I want to say while they are still talking?
- When was the last time I laughed heartily?
- In what situations do I have no sense of humor?
- Do others sometimes judge me as being arrogant, haughty, and proud?
- Do others perceive me as adamant, hard-hearted, and cruel?
- Do I often have cold hands and feet?
- Do I take my duties very, very seriously?
- Am I ready to trust other people with important tasks and decisions?
- Do I sleep deeply, or do I have insomnia?

- How healthy is my heart?
- Am I clear about what is most important to me in life?
- Do I try very hard to always direct what is happening around me?
- Am I sometimes as happy as a small child?
- Who do I love?
- Making love, do I sometimes feel a deep joy?
- Do I sometimes start laughing out of joy while making love?
- Do other people sometimes tell me that my eyes have a sparkle, a shine, a brilliance?

Fire exercises

Looking into the fire

Go into the forest in the afternoon, gather wood, and make a campfire. Sit on the north side of the fire facing the south so that you are looking into the fire. Direct your attention effortlessly and continuously into the flames until you sense that your thoughts have become slower and your consciousness has become filled with the fire. While you are doing this, you can imagine that your thoughts are being devoured by the flames and that your intellect has become one single flame.

Enjoy this state of being for about 15 minutes.

Light meditation

This technique is useful for bringing your mind to rest.

Place a burning candle two to three feet away from you. Look into the flame without blinking. Relax your eyes and sink into a state as I have described above.

Do this exercise once a day for 2–3 weeks if you want to feel an effect on your life.

Mirror meditation

Sit comfortably in front of a mirror and look into your eyes for at least half an hour. Allow your focus to be soft so that you can see your entire face. After a while, you will see other faces and images emerge from under the surface of your own trusted face. This is especially likely to happen if you do this meditation at sundown or by candlelight.

You can also do this exercise with a partner. Sit across from each other, about 5 feet apart, and look into each other's eyes for at least half an hour. You can do this exercise with someone you love; it can also be helpful when you've had a fight in which discussion no longer helps.

Exercises for the Meridians of the Heart, Small Intestine, Pericardium, and San Jiao

Strengthening the Fire-Yin

The Heart posture

This posture speaks for itself. It shows grace and surrender, simplicity and clarity, the ability to be a king as well as a servant.

Enter this posture when you are confused, when disorder reigns in your life, or when you catch yourself under constant stress and have no idea why you don't trust anyone to help you.

Visualize the Heart Meridian, which runs from the middle of the underarm to the inside of the little finger. Intensify your image of this energy flow in your thoughts each time you exhale. Hold this posture for at least three minutes.

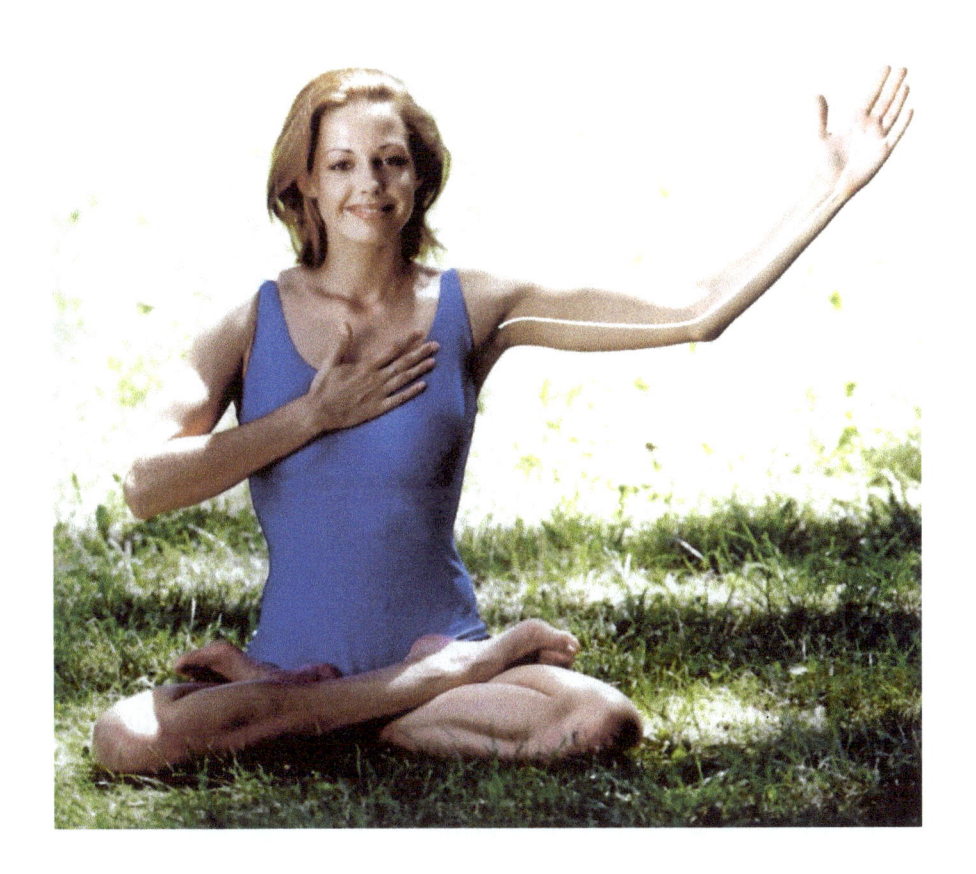

Activating the Heart Meridian

1. Stand with your feet parallel, two feet apart. Hold both arms bent, shoulders relaxed, with the palms of your hands facing upward.

2. Make loose fists.

3. Imagine a reservoir of energy (Qì) just below your navel; this point is called the Hara.

4. Imagine that, with each exhalation, the Qì penetrates into your left fist, and move your fist horizontally forward, as if to punch something. Carry out this movement slowly.

5. With the next inhalation, pull your fist slowly back to its original position.

6. Make the same movement with your right arm.

7. While exhaling, slowly stretch your left fist horizontally to the side. While inhaling, bring it back to its original position.

8. Do the same with your right arm.

9. Repeat this sequence at least five times. When exhaling, imagine that the Qì is bringing about the movement and, when inhaling, that the Qì is returning to the Hara (the pelvis).

Fire • 57

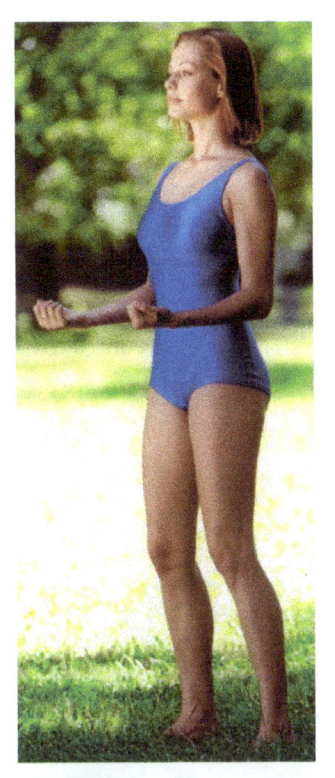

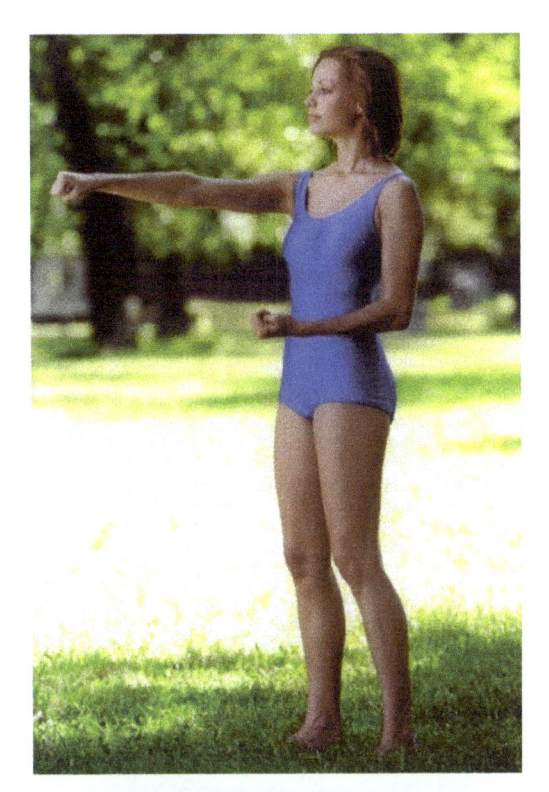

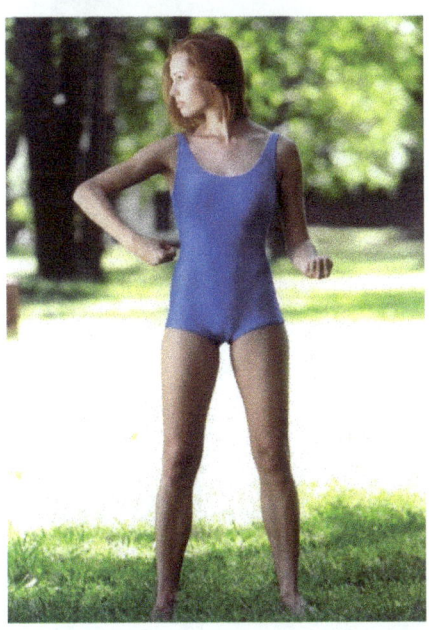

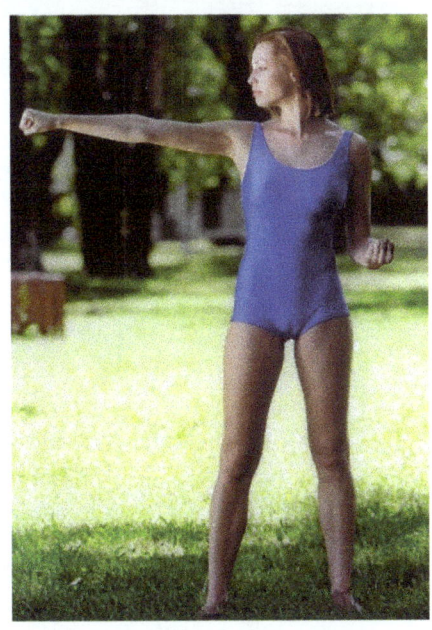

The Pericardium posture

This posture embodies the essence of the Pericardium: openness, warmth, the willingness to give, and the willingness to receive from others. This posture can help you to develop these characteristics.

When you take this posture, visualize the meridian shown in the picture. It flows from the Heart to the hand: It flows one inch away from the sides of the nipples along the surface of the body and runs along the insides of the arms to the last joint of the middle finger. Intensify the energy flow in your imagination while you exhale. Remain in this posture until your hands feel warm and charged.

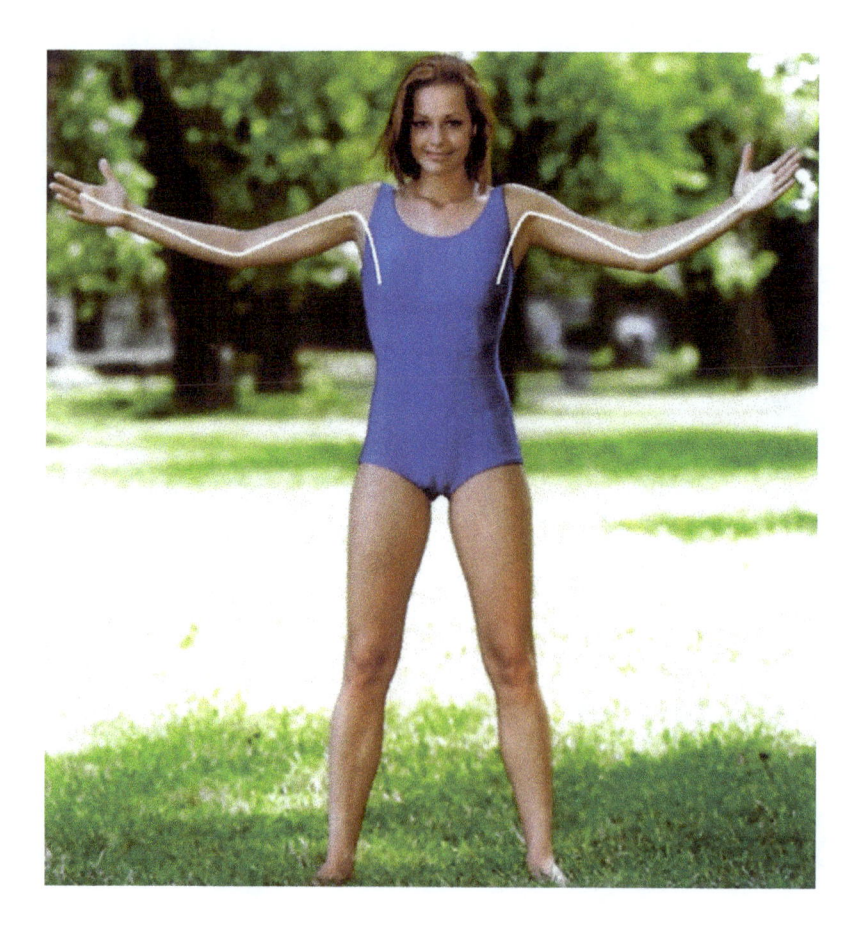

Activating the Pericardium

1. Sit on the floor and bring the soles of your feet together.

2. Rest your hands under your feet with the palms facing up so that the outsides of your ankles are lying on your hands. The point in the middle of the inside of the wrist is Pericardium 7: the Source. It is stimulated through this exercise.

3. While you exhale, stretch the upper part of your body gently in the direction of your feet. While you inhale, return to the original position. Do this exercise for one minute, then remain sitting quietly in this position with your eyes closed and experience the effects of this exercise.

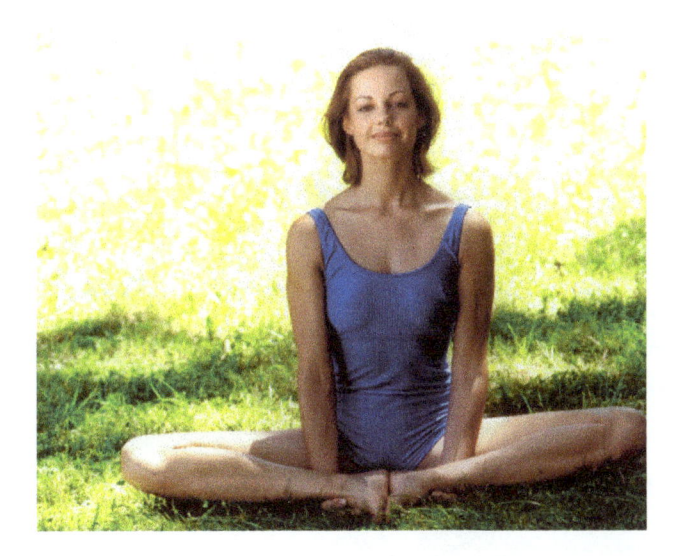

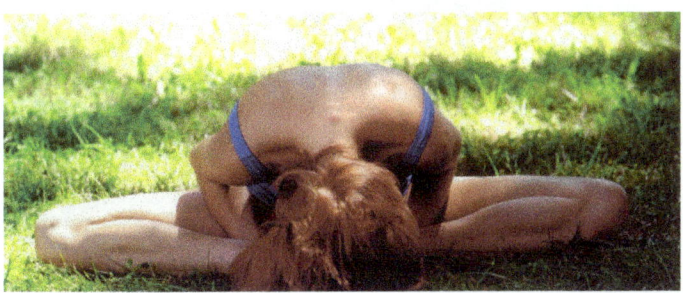

Strengthening the Fire-Yáng

The posture of the Small Intestine

This posture is that of a Kung-Fu fighter using the Qì energy won through assimilation in the Small Intestine for his self-defense. "The organs, Small Intestine, and Bladder eat the Tai Yáng, the highest Yáng, an energy which protects the body from without."

Take the position of the fighter. Tighten your body like a wound-up spring, holding your arm stretched out in front of you. Imagine the Small Intestine Meridian on your right side: The energy flows through this meridian from the tip of your little finger, over your shoulder blade, to your ear. Intensify this flow in your imagination while you inhale. Stay in this posture until you become warm or hot. Then do the exercise on your left side.

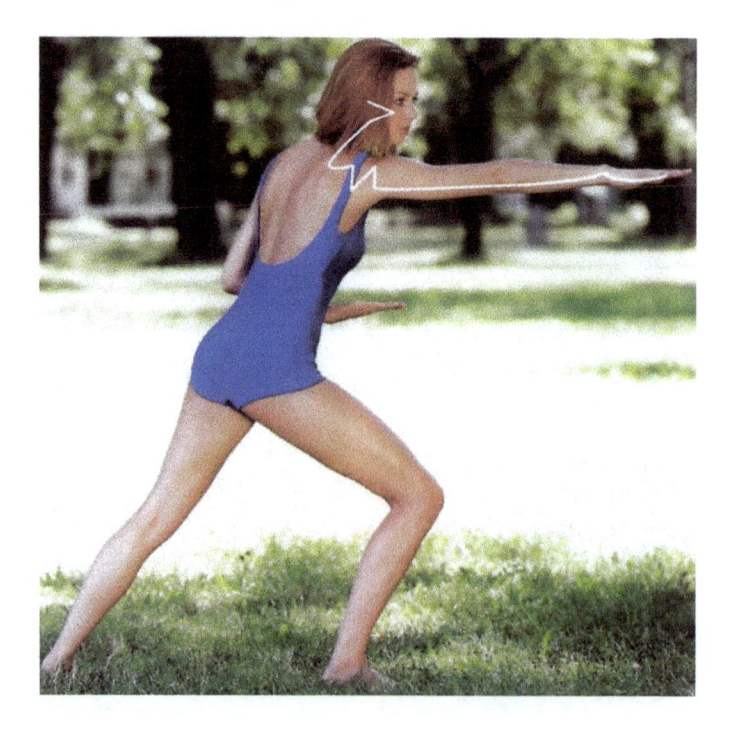

Activating the Small Intestine Meridian

1. Sit on your heels and bring your forehead to the ground. Clasp your hands together behind your back, palms turned toward each other.

2. Inhale and stretch your arms upward and forward so that you feel the tension in your shoulders and shoulder blades. Remain in this posture for about 30 seconds, breathing deeply through your nose.

3. Then stretch your arms a bit farther forward until the tension climaxes.

4. Exhale and let your arms relax on the ground. Feel the effects of this exercise on your body.

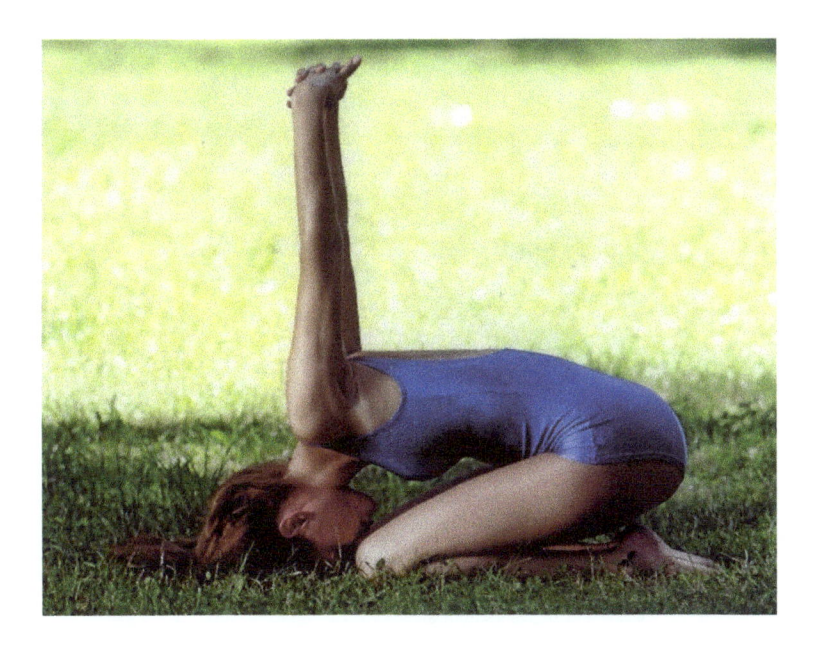

The San Jiao posture

This posture is that of a bird in flight. It expresses the essence of the Triple Warmer: the coordination of the chest, abdomen, and pelvis — of breathing, digestion, and sexuality.

Take the posture of the flying bird and breathe fully and deeply through your mouth. Breathe into your chest and abdomen. Hold your arms stretched out and your head tilted slightly to the side. Visualize the Meridian of the Triple Warmer on your right side, which runs from the ring finger along the arm to the ear, and then to the outside of the eyebrow. Remain in this pose until you become warm or hot. Be careful to remain loose and do not become cramped. Then do the exercise on the left side.

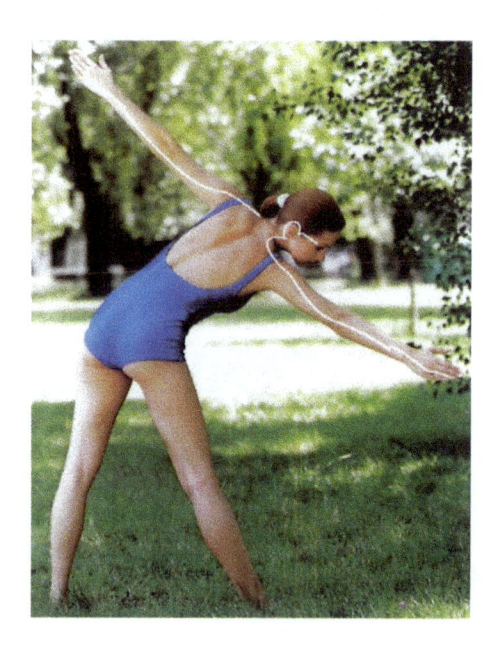

Activating the San Jiao

1. Sit on the ground with your legs stretched out in front of you. Rest your hands behind you on the ground with your fingertips pointing away from you.

2. Raise your pelvis so that your body forms a straight line from your head to your toes.

3. Breathe deeply and regularly for about one minute.

4. Stretch yourself out on the ground keeping your eyes closed, and relax into the pleasant, warm sensation that is created by this exercise.

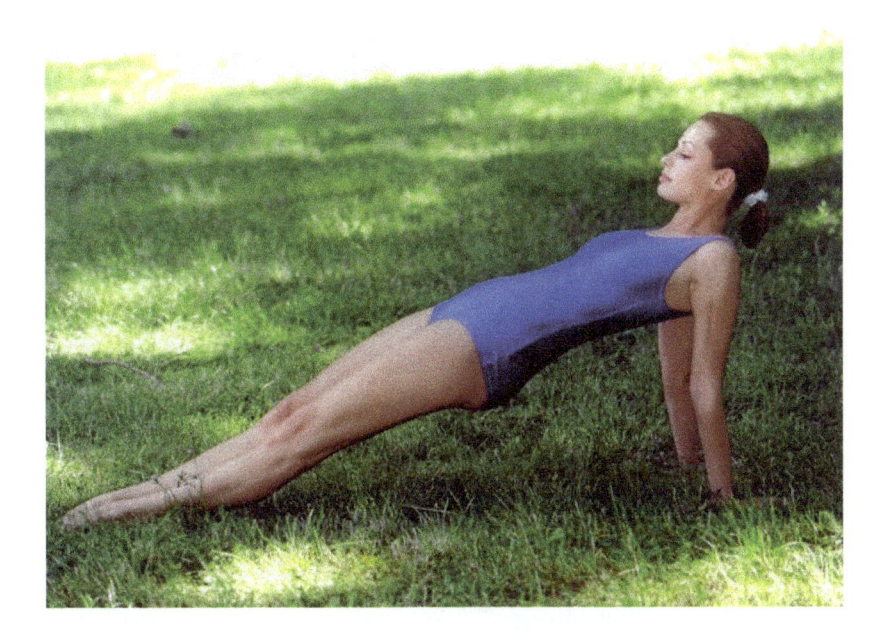

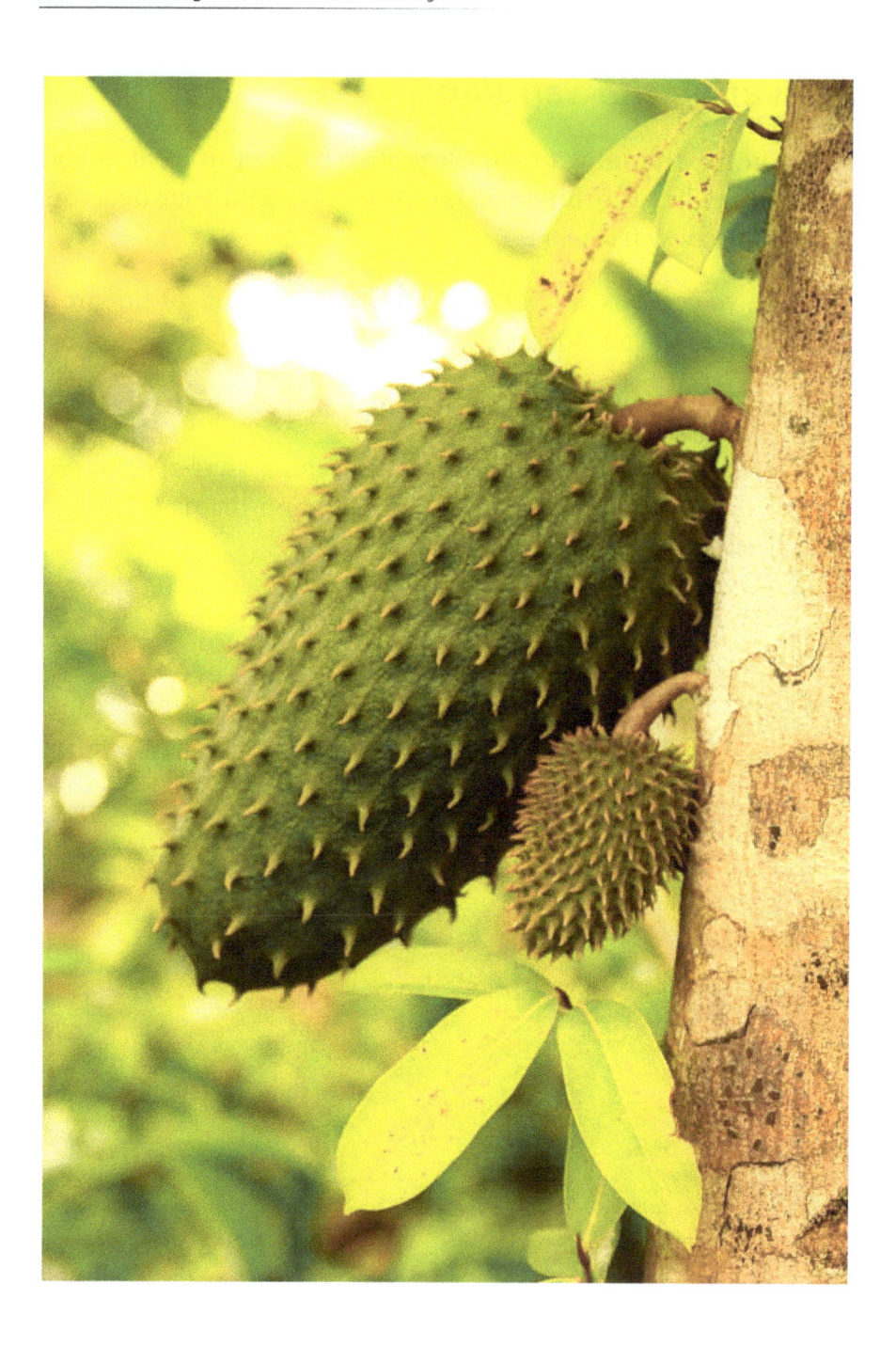

Earth

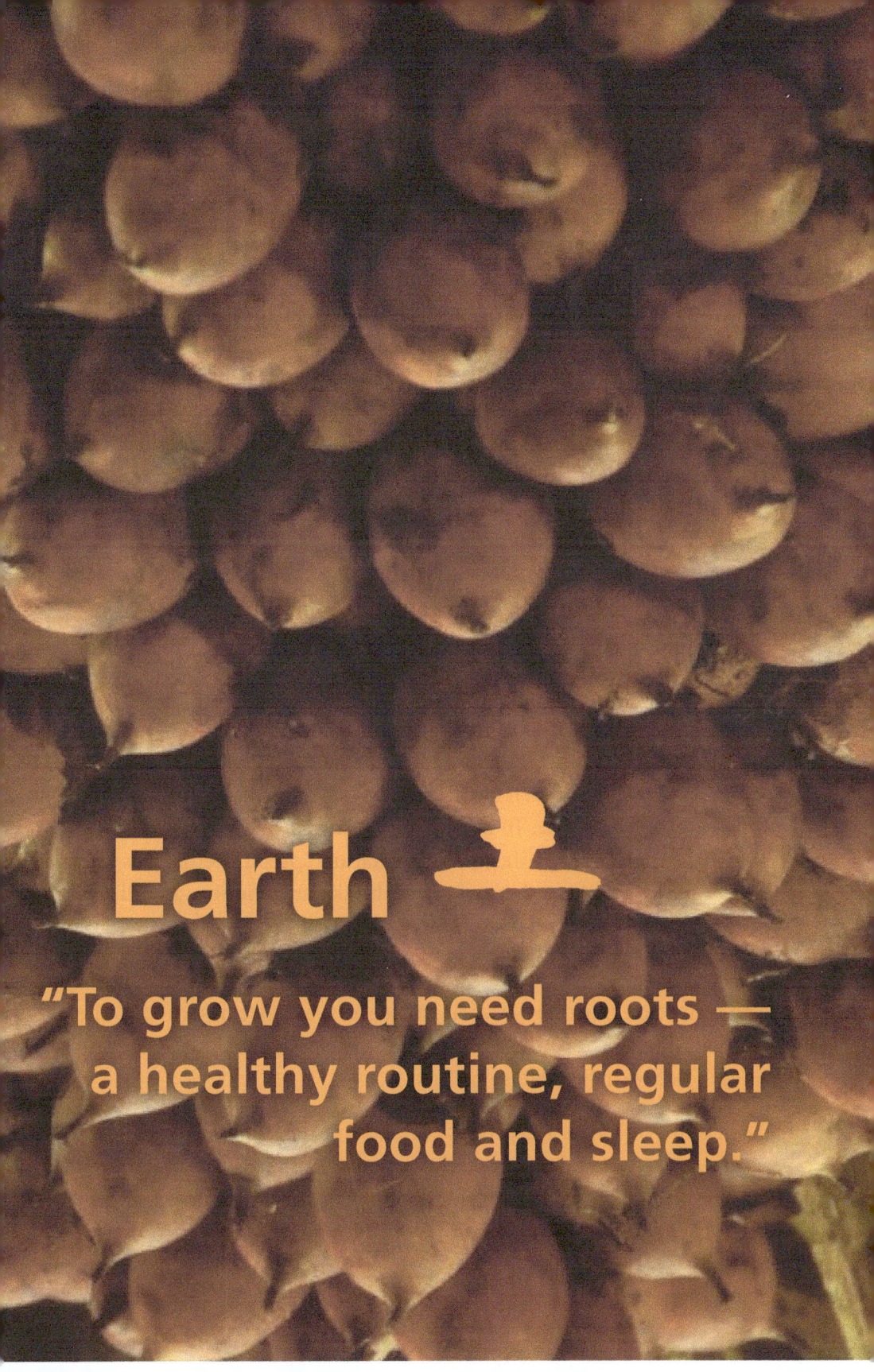

"To grow you need roots —
a healthy routine, regular
food and sleep."

The Element Earth

The season of the year for Earth is late summer, the time when the sun is in the zodiac sign of Virgo. It is the time when nature displays warmth, fullness, and abundance. It is the time when the grains are harvested, and the time of harvest festivals. In farming communities, the fruits of the forest and fields are gathered, sorted out, and dried, and the storage cellars and pantries are filled. An important task during this time of year is the choosing and preparation of foodstuffs that will ensure survival in winter. It is necessary to be concerned that the provisions last for the whole winter. It is the time of gathering and of collecting, as the height of summer with its dance festivals, romance, and pleasures is over, and what is left behind are the nostalgic memories of what was experienced. While in spring a person looks forward to summer, and in summer experiences the pleasures of the present moment, late summer is the time to look back at what was and process it.

The middle is the direction assigned to Earth; it is neither Yin nor Yáng; the direction of its energy is a horizontal, closed circle. Late summer is the time when nature makes the transition from its Yáng phase to its Yin phase. In spring and summer, the powers of light prevail and all the manifestations of nature spread themselves out, grow higher, and turn themselves to the sky and the sun. In fall and winter, the powers of darkness prevail. Nature hides; it draws back inside itself.

The transition periods between the seasons are also assigned to the element Earth. These are moments for looking inside and collecting oneself before a new phase begins.

The colors of Earth are yellow and brown; its climate is moist, as, without water and dampness, the fullness and fertility of the Earth cannot manifest themselves. For Europeans, this allocation does not seem to be very important, as there is enough moisture throughout the year at this latitude. However, in the tropics and subtropics — and large parts of China fall within this area — late summer is the time of the monsoon with its fierce, gushing rainfall and its steamy humidity that follows the glaring heat of the summer and makes the Earth fertile again.

In almost all myths, the Earth plays an important role. The fertility goddesses and Earth goddesses are one symbol in most cultures, bringing the Earth, motherliness, and the sustaining of life together with security and safety, nourishment and fertility, and fullness and generosity. In people, Earth expresses itself through compassion, recognition, sympathy, and a feeling of love and unity with one's environment — through a basic feeling that one is welcome and at home where one is at that moment.

One also finds this feeling in people who quickly gain a sense of well-being in a new environment and who feel accepted by others. This basic feeling gives self-assurance that doesn't need to be proven, an inner security and calmness. In contrast to this, people with a weakness in the Earth element feel insecure, often begging for attention and affection. Underneath this behavior lies the fear that warmth and affection could be taken away or denied. This attitude is often found in people who were not nourished with much love in their early childhood, or who often had to change residences or familiar environments. In psychotherapy today, this behavioral complex is called an "oral character" or "oral fixation."

People with an imbalance in the element Earth often lack compassion; they seem not to enter into relationships with others, and the affairs of others don't seem to touch them very much. A critical stance toward others usually goes hand in hand with this, wherein harsh judgments and low tolerance mask one's own insecurity. With the help of critical remarks, these people are trying to build up their own sense of superiority. Another manifestation of a weakened Earth is self-pity and constant whining about one's own problems.

Such people often play the martyr. A classic example of this is the woman who sacrifices herself for her husband and children, not treating herself to anything. She can moan and point to her destiny as the reason for this.

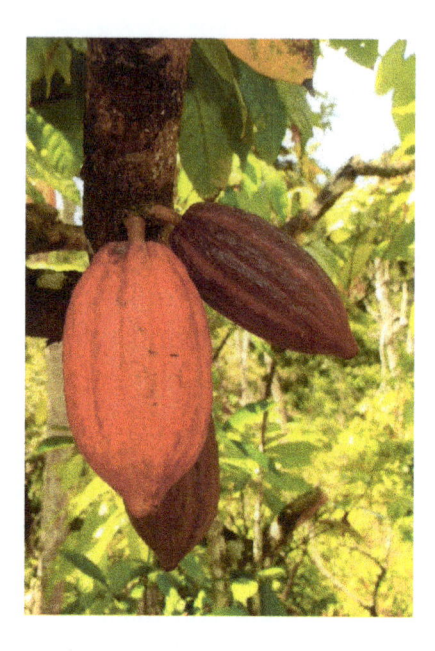

The search for missing security is the driving force and main occupation of people with weak Earth. They look for this security in eating or in smoking, or they are overly affectionate, grasping for love, and constantly looking for the security of motherly love in their relationships. They often hide their fear of abandonment behind a romantic ideal of love and partnership.

A person with a healthy Earth element has an inner abundance from which to give and care for others. Such a person has a sweet scent, just as most fruits have a sweet scent and flavor in late summer when nature displays fullness and abundance. If, however, the Earth element is lacking, it leads to a constant overflow of sticky emotional outbursts and to over-exaggerated generosity, which serves to make others dependent. This behavior is often found in mothers who hinder their children from becoming adults by limiting their responsibilities and not allowing them to make decisions. The tender, lightly sweet scent of the Earth becomes unpleasantly sweet in such people. The natural desire for ripe fruits and grains becomes an addiction to sweet things. The melodic, singing quality that the Earth gives to the voice becomes a whining, moaning sing-song.

Only where there is inner security is there a purpose for oneself, and a reality in which fullness and abundance are possible. Only when possessing this fullness is a person able to love and care for others. Without this inner wealth, the pleasant, sweet quality of the Earth turns into an outer show — a mask covering one's own emptiness.

The elemental spirit of Earth is called Yì. Its homes are the Spleen and Pancreas, the Yin organs of Earth. Its qualities are logical thinking and a rational intellect, the ability to be critical, the ability to think things over, and a good memory. Other characteristics are worrying about a thousand and one things or brooding over the past and indulging in reminiscences. On a mental level, the effect of Earth can be seen in the same concepts and categories that are used to label the period of late summer: gathering, processing, selecting, mental nourishment, survival, and gaining the wisdom that gives us the security to deal with difficult situations in life.

The word "intellect" comes from the Latin verb *legere*, which means "to read" and "to gather." An intellectual reads a lot, broods over things, gathers information in the Brain, stores it, and processes it if the intellect has enough Fire, enough independence, to be able to digest and assimilate the gathered ideas.

The greed for knowledge and the latest news, and an addiction to reading, can be traced to an overstimulated Spleen. Above all, this is displayed in an accumulation of knowledge about detailed areas of human life — in the type of knowledge that specialists have, concentrated without seeing the connection to the bigger picture.

A Shí state, or Fullness, of the Spleen is also found in people who cannot stop thinking — who have to think through and consider everything, whose intellect is constantly caught in an inner monologue. A Shí state of the Spleen can also be found in one-sided advocates of science and reason, in people who judge and reject every other way of looking at things. Such people try to compensate for a deficit in Earth energy by mentally clinging to an apparent security in the logical verification of things.

Other symptoms of a Shí state of the Spleen are compulsive behavior, fixed ideas, obsessions, and a passion for collecting. If the person is a collector, the degree of imbalance can be recognized in whether that person gathers useful and valuable objects, for example, paintings or antiques or completely absurd objects that have become an obsession.

One can also see different forms and levels of obsession. In our culture, many people are obsessed with an idea or a way of life: work, status, power, success, and money. In ancient China, one spoke more commonly of an obsession in relation to being possessed by demons and spirits, although it is actually the same phenomenon. An idea or a demon gets the upper hand in a person's mind to such an extent that this person becomes blind to the variety of life, losing contact with the body, feelings, and self.

All people have an individually varying supply of elemental energies available to express themselves on the physical, emotional, and mental levels. For instance, if a person uses up a large portion of Earth energy for taking in nourishment and digestion, there won't be much energy left over for thought and reflection. If a person uses up a large portion of Earth energy through intellectual work, then there will be a deficit on the organic and emotional levels. He/she will have little compassion because his/her intellect is so occupied with other things. And, if you use up a lot of your Earth energy through your thinking process, there probably will be sooner or later a deficit of Earth energy on the physical level, leading to allergies, or menstrual problems, or stomach ulcers and metabolic disorders.

The Yin organ of Earth is commonly called the Spleen. As I mentioned in the chapter on the organs, Chinese medicine has a more energetic approach to the body and that is why organs are defined in a different way. On the physical level, the Spleen consists of two main systems or "organs" in the body: first, the exocrinic part of the Pancreas and, second, the Reticulo-Endothelial System (RES), a network of reticular connective tissue and endothelium that forms various anatomical structures in the body.

The exocrinic part of the Pancreas produces preliminary digestive enzymes which enter the digestive tract in the middle of the duodenum. Their function is the breakdown of proteins, fats, and carbohydrates. They become highly activated in the duodenum and Small Intestine and finish where the digestive process begins in the mouth and Stomach.

In the Chinese tradition, the duodenum and the first six inches of the Small Intestine are considered part of the Stomach. This is important because a large part of the absorption of nutrients takes place in the first six inches of the Small Intestine. Consequently, one can understand why the Chinese attribute the digestion of food and nourishment of the body to the Earth organs and, only to a lesser extent, to the Small Intestine.

RES is a medical term that describes, on one hand, the lymphatic tissues and organs: the Spleen, Lymph Nodes, Lymphatic Vessels, Tonsils, Appendix, and Thymus. On the other hand, the RES also includes the red Bone Marrow, the copper star cells of the Liver, and the mucus membranes of the Intestine with its large number of Lymph Follicles.

The major tasks of the lymphatic system can be summarized as follows:

1. Draining — the transport of "excess" water from the tissue back into the blood.

2. Absorption of fat from the Intestine to the intestinal Lymphatic Vessels.

3. Generation of lymphocytes (the essential part of the body's immune system) in the Bone Marrow, Lymph Nodes, and Spleen.

4. Storage and breakdown of red blood cells in the Spleen.

If one ties together the above descriptions of the functions of the Pancreas and RES, one can see a clear picture of the functions of the Earth organs according to traditional view: The Spleen is the mother organ of the physical body. The Spleen regulates the distribution of water and blood. It is the nourisher of the body. The organic tissues that are assigned to Earth are the connective tissue, fat tissue, and muscle fibers. Its Yáng organ is the Stomach, and its sensory organ the mouth, especially the lips and the mouth cavity. It communicates to the outer world through taste and touch. Its bodily fluids are saliva and lymph.

The main functions of the Earth organs are nourishment and maintenance of the body. In contrast to our understanding, the Chinese notion of "nourishment" refers to not only providing nutrients but also providing oxygen via the erythrocytes to every cell in the body: The erythrocytes — or red blood cells — are formed in the red Bone Marrow which belongs to the Spleen. That is why the ancient texts emphasized the following: "The Spleen regulates the blood."

Another important aspect of maintaining the body´s unscathedness is the work of the immune system, whose components belong to the Spleen: The red Bone Marrow generates the B-lymphocytes which produce antibodies, and the lymphatic organs — the main lymphatic organs are the Lymph Glands and the Spleen — generate the T-lymphocytes which are programmed to fight specific antigens.

As the lymphatic vessels transport fluids from the tissue to the bloodstream, the Spleen regulates the distribution of water in the body in general, especially the tone of the skin. As long as our Spleen is vital and strong, we radiate youth and health.

Since the Earth organs nourish and maintain the body, the Spleen is seen not only as the mother of the physical body but also as the organ responsible for fertility, pregnancy, and birth, in conjunction with the Kidney and the Uterus. The breasts are assigned to the element Earth, whereas the Uterus is considered an extraordinary organ.

Out of this composition, the clinical meaning of the Spleen and Stomach Meridians becomes clear. An imbalance results in disorders including illnesses of the digestive system, such as indigestion, gastritis, stomach and duodenal ulcers, incomplete digestion, pancreatitis, diarrhea, and constipation; illnesses of the immune system, such as allergies, autoimmune diseases (in which Wood also plays a part), immune deficiencies, a disposition toward illness, menstrual problems, infertility, pain and swelling of the breasts (especially in connection with the menses), inflammation of the mammary glands, problems with lactating, skin diseases, edema, and swelling; and, finally, illnesses of the Lymph Nodes and Lymphatic Vessels.

Disturbances in the rhythm of the human organism point to an imbalance in the element Earth. The rhythms of sleeping and waking, of appetite and digestion, and of breathing, as well as the menstrual cycle and the rhythm of physical, spiritual, and mental activity, are all determined by the revolution of the earth on its axis. They follow the rhythm of day and night, the cycle of the moon and the tides, and the changing of the seasons. Since the moon is so closely connected to the rhythms of the earth, in many cultures it is assigned to Earth and is seen as the symbol for fertility and birth. However, it is also often assigned to Water, as its revolution affects the tides. The Earth plays a central role in the Chinese way of thinking. In the original diagrams of the Five Elements, Earth is portrayed in the center, and the elements Water, Wood, Fire, and Metal and the four directions arrange themselves around it. In ancient China, there were medical and spiritual schools based on handling every physical and spiritual complaint by bringing the element Earth into balance. They attained this through an extensive, practical knowledge about the powers of the elements in various foods, through the use of herbs and extracts of herbs, through massage and acupuncture of the Stomach and Spleen–Pancreas Meridians, and through special mental and physical exercises to strengthen the Earth energy in a person's disposition.

Our language includes many ways to express our connection with Earth: "standing with both feet on the ground," "mother earth," "to not feel the ground under one's feet," and many more. The Earth is our central, physical reality from the moment we begin our lives in the womb until we return to the Earth. Our sense of reality is based on the strength of the Earth element in us. How we present ourselves, whether we have both feet on the ground, whether we feel "at home" and secure in our lives, whether we feel comfortable in our skin, and whether we radiate and look healthy and vital all depend on our connection to Earth.

Mental and Physical Exercises to Strengthen the Earth

Clarifying questions

Proceed with the questions as you have done previously.

- Do I feel comfortable in my surroundings most of the time?
- Do I feel comfortable in my skin?
- Do I generally feel loved and accepted by the people around me, or do I feel unloved and misunderstood?
- Do I get the attention I want?
- Am I a compassionate person?
- Do other people come to me to tell me their worries and problems, or am I occupied most of the time with my own affairs?
- Am I more likely to be good-natured or demanding?
- Am I possessive in a love relationship?
- Do I have a rigid idea of how my relationship with my partner should be?
- Do I try to control my partner or to change his or her ways?
- Can I be happy about how my partner is?
- Do I have a strong, healthy constitution, or am I often sick?
- Do I suffer from allergies?
- Do I sleep deeply and have a healthy appetite and a glowing appearance?

- Do I like to eat, and do I take pleasure in it?
- Do I have a healthy stomach?
- Am I preoccupied with my diet, eating habits, and nourishment ideals?
- Do I eat my meals with regularity?
- Do I sometimes have a feeling of fullness in my abdomen after I eat?
- Do I have a firm or a flabby body?
- Am I overly critical of myself or others?

Earth exercises

Grounding yourself

It is best to do this exercise in the forest, on a lawn, or on the beach. However, it can also be done on a blanket in your room. A good time for this exercise is in the afternoon or early evening.

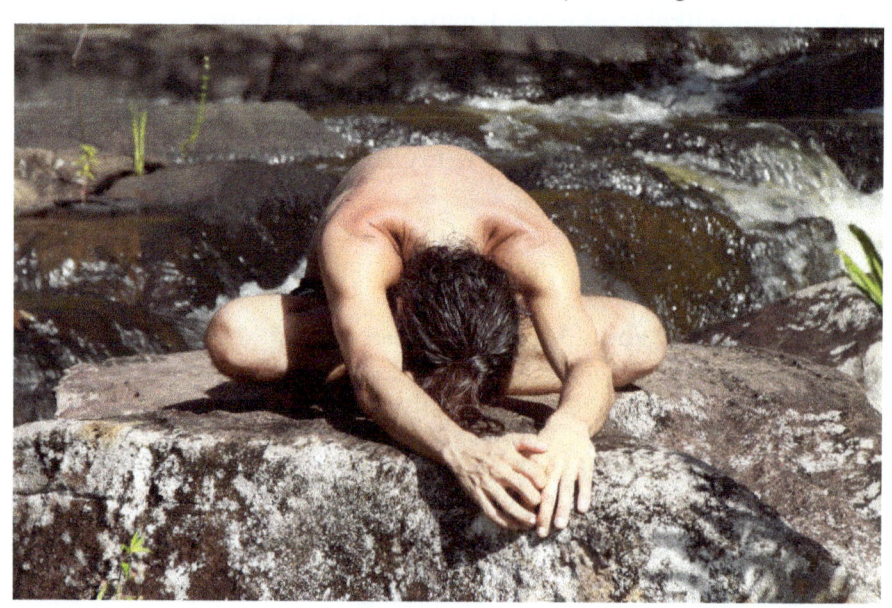

Lie on your stomach and stretch yourself out like a cat. Then let yourself sink into the ground. Imagine that you are composed of Earth — heavy and still.

Remain in this position for at least 15 minutes. To concentrate your thoughts, use the mantra "Yì." If you want to strengthen the power in your Hara, place a tennis ball underneath your abdomen, about two finger-widths below your belly button. With every breath, relax your abdomen more and more.

Compassion

Look for someone around you who needs attention. Take two hours of your time to be with him or her. Find out what this person needs and what makes him or her happy.

Eating consciously

Prepare your own meals for a week. Prepare food that tastes good, is easy to digest, and gives you strength. Enjoy it! Invite someone to eat with you occasionally.

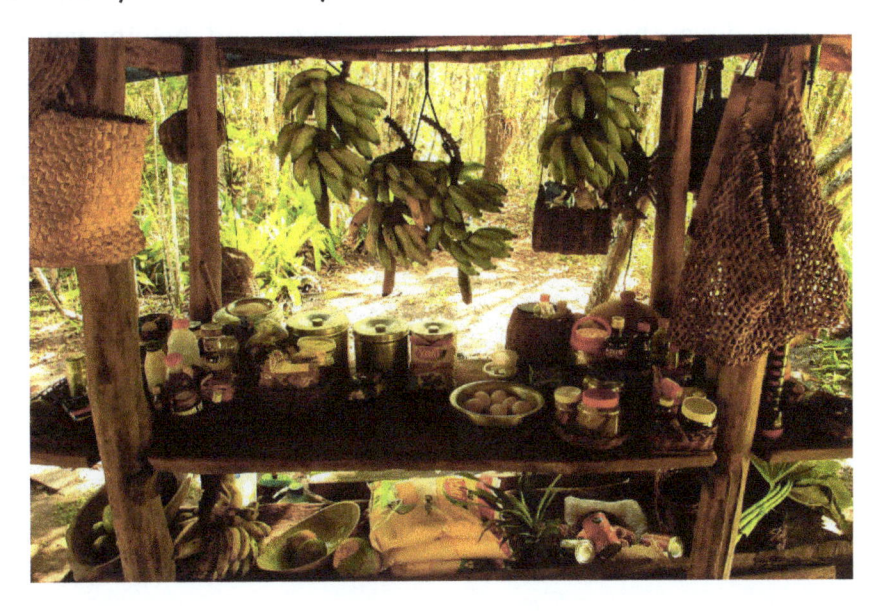

Exercises for the Stomach and Spleen Meridians

Strengthening the Earth-Yáng

The Stomach posture

This posture represents the circle — the circle being the symbol of Earth.

Hold this posture for a minute. Breathe regularly through your mouth, which should be slightly open. Make sure that the palm of your upper hand is facing the ceiling and that the palm of your lower hand is facing the ground. Visualize the Stomach Meridian first only on the right side, on the side of your raised arm. The energy flows through the meridian from a point under your right eye, down your face and neck, to the middle of your right clavicle. From there, the meridian runs down across the chest to your right nipple and further down over the abdomen to the pubic bone. There, the meridian crosses the groin to the outside and runs along the front of the leg, down to the tip of the second toe. Imagine a yellow stream of energy that runs down this meridian and into the ground, helping you to feel the ground underneath your feet more intensely.

After a minute, exhale and stretch your right hand as far up as you can and your left hand as far down as you can. Then take the posture for the left side and visualize the left Stomach Meridian.

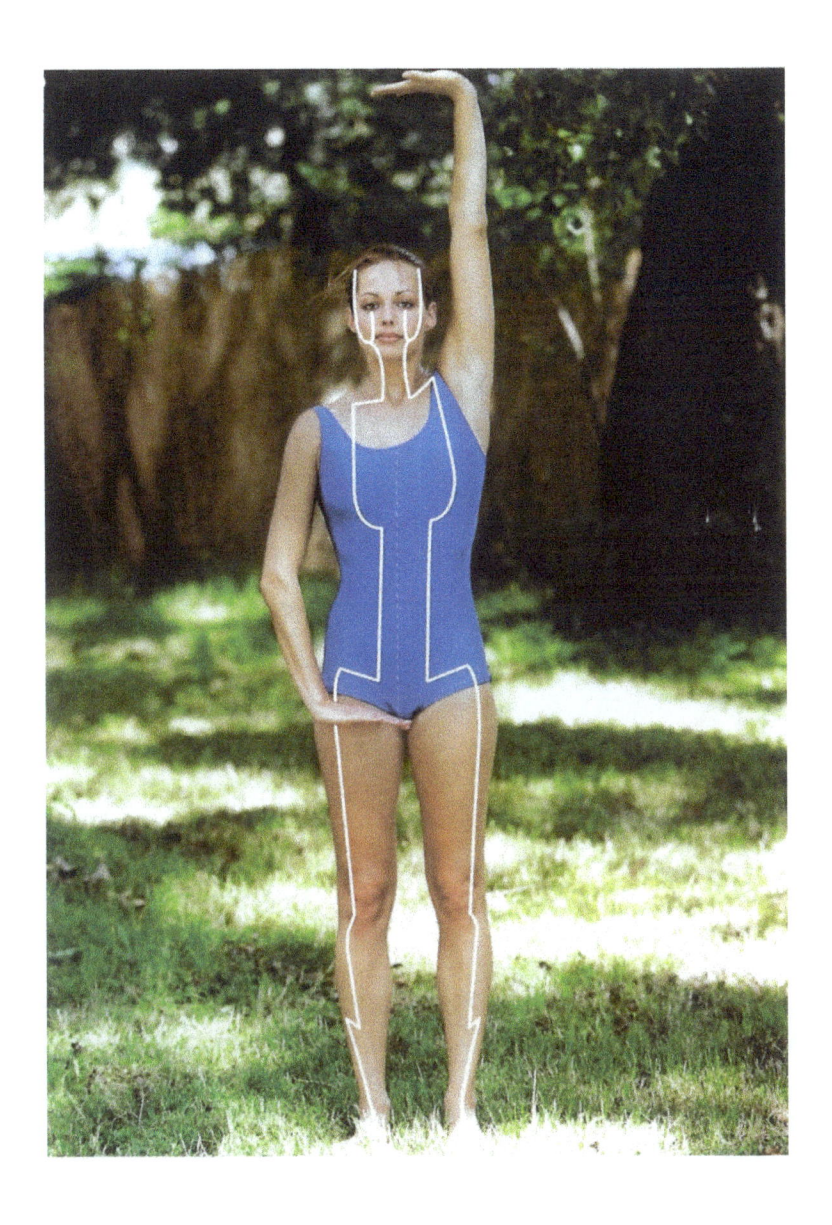

Activating the Stomach Meridian

Sit on the ground with your legs bent under you so that your feet are on either side of your hips. Lower the upper part of your body slowly backward until you feel a tension in your thighs. If you are able, lie for half a minute with your back on the ground and breathe deeply in and out.

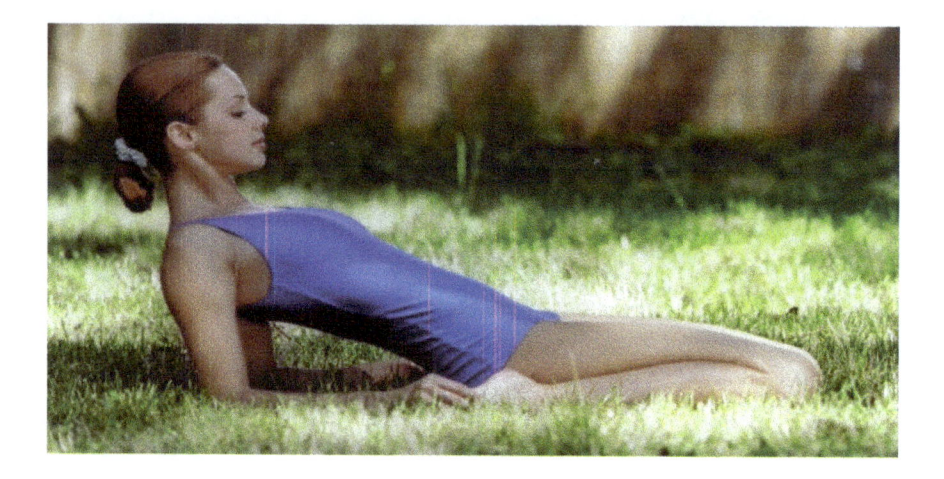

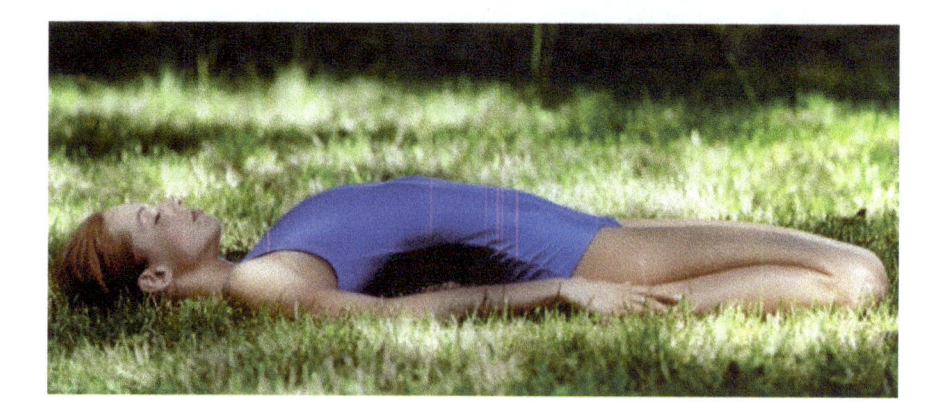

Strengthening the Earth-Yin

The Spleen posture

This posture expresses security, being grounded, and stability — essential qualities of the Spleen energy.

Hold this posture for at least a minute. The distance between your feet should be big enough to allow you to easily let your pelvis sink down. Breathe regularly through your mouth, which should be slightly open. Slowly turn your torso to the right, then to the left, then again to the right, and so on.

The Qì flows through this meridian from the big toe, up the inside of the leg to the groin and to the abdomen, from there further to the breast, and to just before the armpit. Then the meridian runs a bit farther down to its endpoint, which is in the middle of the flank. Imagine that you pull the Qì up through the meridian to its endpoint with every inhalation.

While you turn your torso to the right, visualize the left Spleen Meridian with every inhalation. While you exhale, turn your torso back to its original position. While you are turning to the left, visualize the right Spleen Meridian with every inhalation.

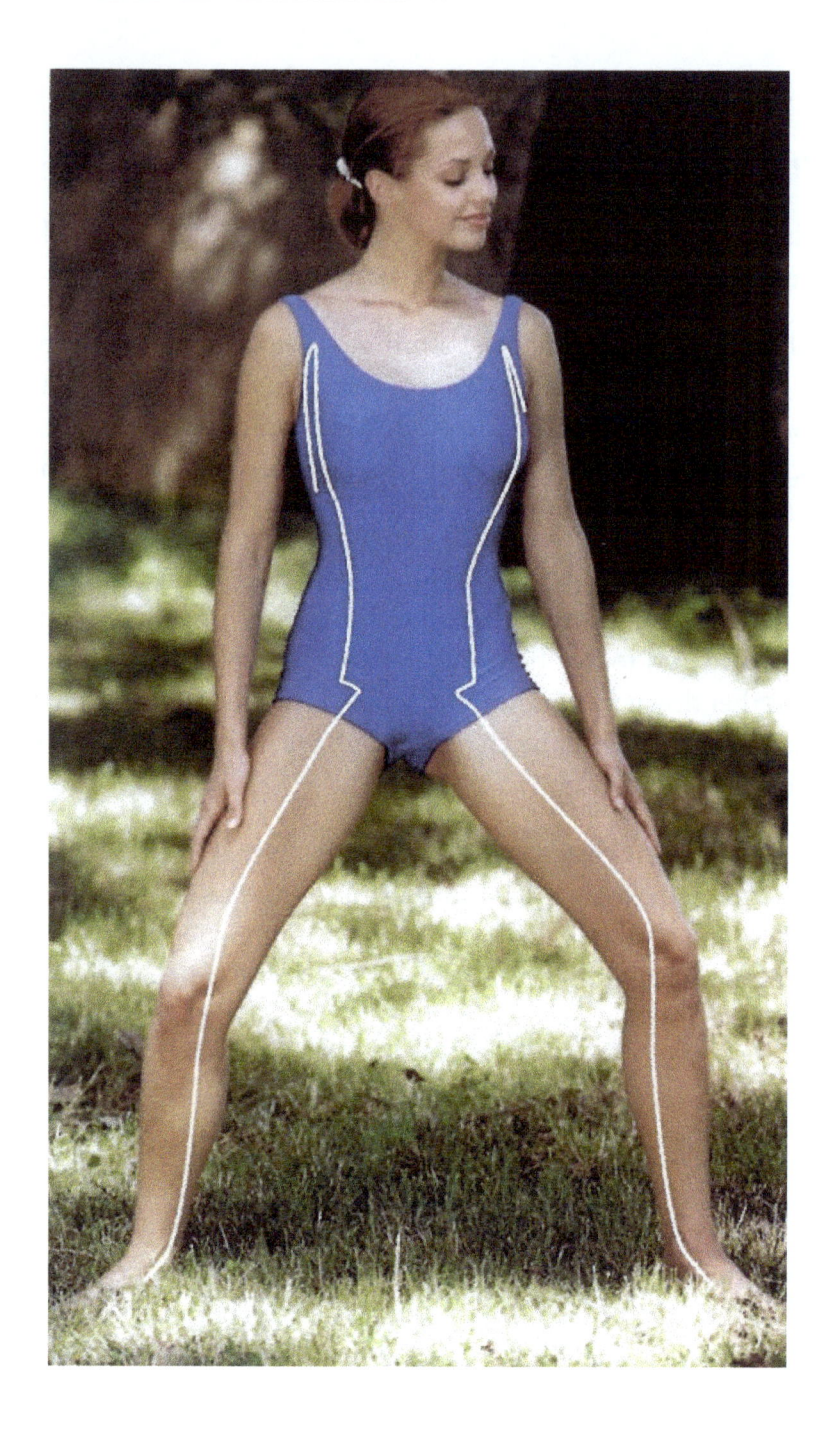

Activating the Spleen Meridian

1. Lie on your stomach with your hands underneath your body so that your fists are under your groin.

2. Breathe in and raise your stretched legs as far as possible off the ground. Remain in this position for half a minute, breathing deeply in and out.

3. While breathing out, lower your legs slowly to the ground and let your arms relax next to your body. Be careful that no tension remains in the small of your back.

4. Lie for another minute on your stomach and imagine that your body is filled with the color yellow.

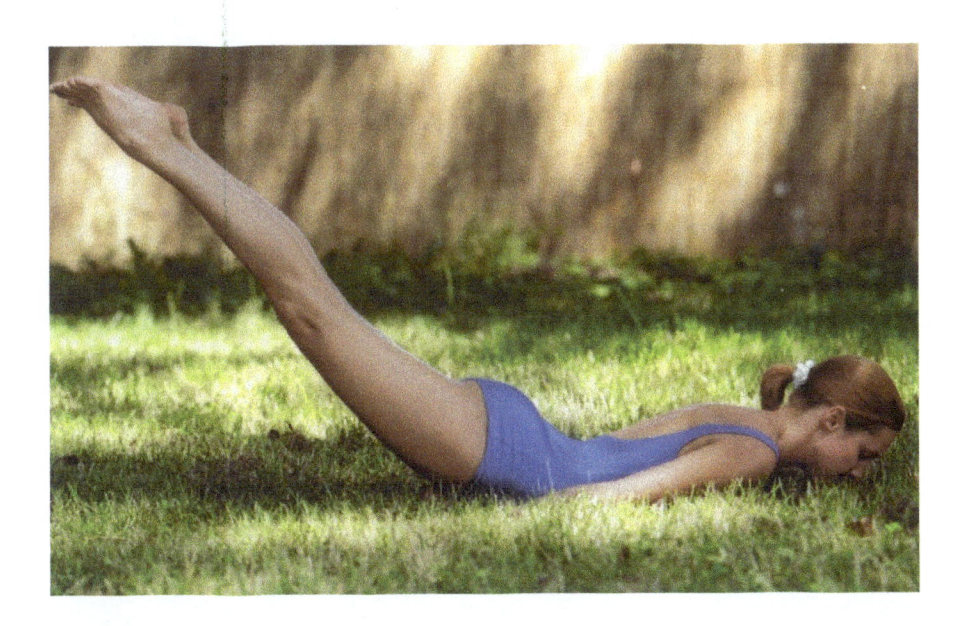

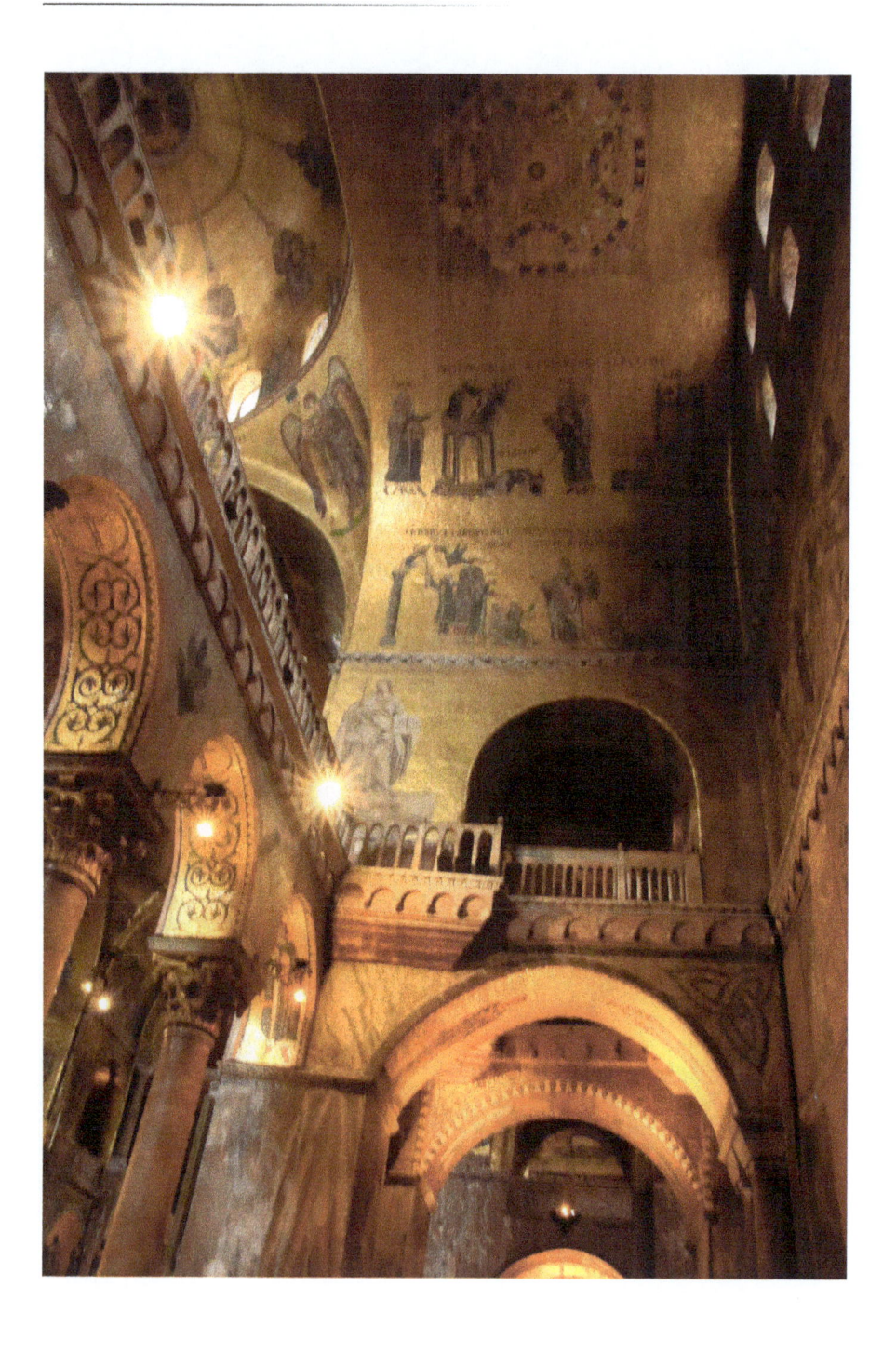

Metal 金

"You waste your life, if you do not daily concentrate on the essential.
To concentrate on the essential, you have to cut loose from unhealthy habits and false friends."

The Element Metal

Fall depicts the essence of Metal: concentration and condensation; the energy is directed within. The withering of plants and the withdrawal of the life force that we experience in fall is the exact opposite of the expansive energy of spring. Metal is the opposite of Wood. Just as Wood is called the "young Yáng," Metal embodies the "young Yin." Its direction is the west; its climate is dry; its time of day is evening.

The four elements of Western tradition are earth, air, fire, and water. In ancient Greek culture, there was originally a fifth element — spirit or ether — whose characteristics are found not only in Wood and Fire but also in Metal. Metal corresponds to the Greek element of air, although it has additional meanings. The names of some points on the Lung Meridian show the relationship to air — for example, Lung 2, "The Gate to the Clouds," and Lung 3, "Palace of Heaven" — but the meanings of most of the names go deeper, as the essence of the element Metal is structure, distance, depth, and dimension. This expresses itself in names, such as "Large Abyss" (Lu 9), "Missing Order" (Lu 7), and "Oblique Junction" (LI 6).

Metal symbolizes concentrated energy, an essence that keeps the universe together. Power sites in nature were used by ancient cultures for ritual purposes. They built their temples and churches and even magnificent structures such as the Cheops Pyramid and Stonehenge in special places on the earth where invisible yet perceptible energy fields inspire awe and prayer. Power sites and the network of energy lines on the surface of the earth are ascribed to the Metal element.

The trace elements and minerals of the earth are assigned to Metal; without them, growth would be impossible, to mention the earth's ability to produce nutrients. Earth is the mother; Metal is the father and is responsible for structure, support, and concentration on what is essential. When these two come together, the possibility for birth and growth, in the sense of the element Wood, comes to be.

The Yin organ of Metal are the Lungs; the Yáng organ is the Large Intestine. In the Chinese tradition, the Lungs were compared to the first minister of state — the high priest who fulfilled sacred functions which were necessary for the maintenance of order in the community. The Lungs "receive the life energy, the Qì of heaven;" the Large Intestine is "the eliminator of waste." In this, the two basic functions of the element Metal can be seen: receiving and releasing the basic forms of energy transfer with our environment.

In the Hindu tradition, the essence of the breath is called the "life energy," or Prana, a term that is similar to the Chinese Qì. Wilhelm Reich discovered this life energy in his research and called it "Orgone." Modern particle physics uses the term "quantum fields."

Most spiritual traditions use concentration and control of the breath as a meditation technique. In such traditions, the breath is viewed as our connection to the universe and our conscious use of it as a means to live in harmony with heaven and earth. This is because the breath assumes the middle position between our conscious and unconscious life; the rhythm of the breath is controlled from the center of the autonomic nervous system, yet it can be consciously controlled by any person. Through this, the awareness of the breath is the first, most important step for most people in becoming conscious of the otherwise unconscious processes of the organs.

With every exhalation, the Lungs fulfill the most important eliminatory function of the body: the release of carbon dioxide created in the respiratory process. Exhaling means becoming free of toxic substances and creating space for new energy production. One can differentiate between two styles of breathing. One type of person breathes in too much and breathes out too little. They strut around with inflated chests, hold on tightly to what they have, and are often incapable of letting go and relaxing. The other type breathes out more than in. Their chests are collapsed, they suffer from a constant lack of energy, and they constantly look needy, although they have oxygen right in front of their noses.

The double function of the breath — the energetic charge and discharge — is a principle found all over the cosmos. It is the principle of the pulse, the change from expansion to contraction. This principle is found in the behavior of galaxies as well as in the behavior of amoebas and other one-celled organisms. Although concentration is the basic movement of Metal, this does not contradict the principle of pulse or breathing because it is only by rhythmic change from tension to relaxation that a concentration of energy can develop. Rhythm is a basic term for Metal. A rhythmic breathing that fully unfolds itself makes the pulse of life in us possible and gives us the power to stay in touch with our environment.

While the Lungs "receive the life energy, the Qì of heaven," the Large Intestine is "the eliminator of waste." In this, the two basic functions of the element Metal can be seen: receiving and releasing, the basic forms of energy transfer with our environment.

It is thus clear that the element Metal represents our relationship to the universe — our "connection to heaven." The complementary abilities of receiving and excreting or letting go form the basis of mental and physical health. If the ability to receive is poorly developed, the organism suffers from a deficiency; it is cut off. If the ability to let go is not developed, the organism will become constipated and will stagnate. This is why the Large Intestine is as important as the Lungs for our "connection to heaven" — heaven being a synonym for the mental and spiritual world. Only if we can let go of mental waste and obsolete mind patterns are we able to grasp fresh ideas and think new thoughts. This is why the functioning of the Large Intestine, on the mental level, means the power of discernment and clarity of thought.

A sign of an imbalance in Metal is an inadequate bond to the environment. People with such an imbalance are often lonely and withdrawn. They seem hard, cold, and isolated from their surroundings, and they show little feeling. Others are ambitious, have high ideals, and strive for something that they can never get. Still others are religious in a fixed and dogmatic way. They have a strong desire to get to heaven. They know many techniques to purify themselves, and they try to convert others to their beliefs and to a pure life. They are, however, incapable of letting themselves go enough to receive the spiritual quality of the essence of Metal. This behavior is understandable when one remembers that the Lungs and Large Intestine make up the most important eliminatory systems in the body and that, with too little excretion and too shallow breathing, the desire for inner and outer purification becomes very great. Cleanliness and hygiene fanatics, extreme proponents of macrobiotics, and religious dogmatists are often compensating for their disturbance in Metal with such behavior.

In the fall, the people in simple farming communities are thinking about how they will survive the winter. On gloomy days, they perhaps worry about the future. An imbalance in Metal is also revealed by a person's exaggerated worry about the future. With a disturbance in Metal, one also finds a pessimistic attitude toward life, a hopelessness. However, if Metal is healthy, then trust in life, optimism, and a positive assessment of the future prevail.

The feeling that corresponds to the fall is sadness. It is the sadness that fills us when we have to take leave of something that has become precious and dear to us. One finds this feeling exaggerated in people who are not able to let go of something that they can never get back A general sadness can also develop as a result of a weak bond to the world or a lack of vitality and life energy-insufficient Qì. We can also feel sad about things that have not yet happened when we realize that we have not taken advantage of our opportunities.

The tissue that corresponds to Metal is the skin. Here, one can also see the basic principles of this element. The skin is an important eliminatory and breathing organ. We are constantly in touch with our environment through our skin. It responds to the accumulation of waste products by developing various skin diseases and reacting to some environmental stimuli through allergies. We show our attitudes toward other people by allowing them to touch us or by avoiding contact with them. We are in touch with nature only as long as we enjoy the sensation of the coolness of the water and the wind, the warmth of the sun, the softness or roughness of the earth, and the tenderness of the leaves and plants on our skin.

The sensory organ of Metal is the nose. A limited or nonexistent sense of smell points to an imbalance in Metal. The properties of smell are closely connected to the elemental spirit of Metal, called Po. With Po, the Chinese designate the animal instinct that gives us the ability to smell danger, lets us sense how other people are thinking and feeling about us, and allows us to foresee future events. Our sense of smell makes it possible for us to differentiate between foods, surroundings, and people that may be good or bad for us. It allows us to differentiate between the various scents of flowers and plants. We instinctively reject a person whose smell we do not like, while we feel attracted to a person who smells pleasant, whose fragrance entices us.

White is the color assigned to Metal. Most of the time, a white complexion expresses a lack of the Fire element in the personality, a lack of warmth. While Metal is characterized by the striving for intellectual quality, with a deficit in Fire this often turns into a rigid outlook, an intolerant Puritanism, or a religious fanaticism. This type of spirituality lacks enthusiasm, warmth, and spontaneity, characteristics typical of many religions.

It seems to be difficult to live with the power of Metal. On the one hand, the core of Metal is concentration, letting go, grief, going within, and leaving the world. On the other hand, it is the connection to our environment, the connection to our vitality, and the connection to heaven. Often, we have to withdraw in order to perceive a deeper connection that is not visible in our day-to-day lives. Only when we let go of what was can the circle be completed. Only when we let go can a space be created in which the old can die and the new can be born. It is important to remove the outer form so that the essence can reveal itself. It is important to let go without giving up, without losing trust. This is how a retreat from the world becomes a retreat into the essential world.

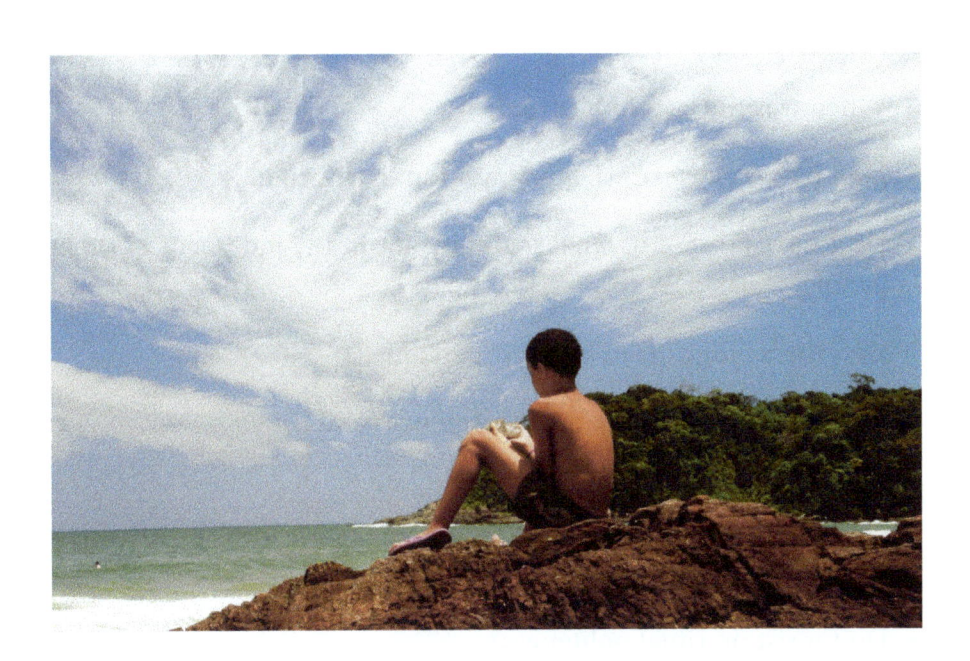

Mental and Physical Exercises to Refine Metal

Clarifying questions

Proceed with the questions as you have done previously.

- How do I feel in fall?

- How do I let go of people or things that have become valuable or dear to me?

- Can I let go of what is gone forever and not surrender myself to false hopes?

- Is it easy for me to withdraw and to concentrate on myself?

- How do I feel when I am alone?

- When was the last time I grieved deeply?

- When was the last time I cried?

- Do I have a sense of what is important in my life?

- Do I have a sense of what is important in my judgment of other people?

- Do others judge me to be a fair person?

- Am I able to clearly formulate sentences and use words skillfully?

- Do I stand on ceremonies and advocate formalities and attention to technicalities?

- Do I insist on ritual politeness?

- Is my behavior sometimes cold and chilly?
- Do I frequently turn down and reject other people?
- Can I smell danger when it is in the air?
- Do I perceive many different smells?
- Do I often have a cold or a flu?
- Do I have a chronic sinus infection?
- Do I tend to strangle feelings by thinking?
- Do I often suffer from bronchitis?
- Have I ever had pneumonia?
- Do I easily get out of breath when I do something strenuous?

Metal exercises

Rhythm of the breath and personality

Dance to music you like for 15 minutes. Then lie stretched out on your back. Observe the natural rhythm of your breath without influencing it in any way. Establish what type of breather you are: Do you exhale more than you inhale (do you have a collapsed, flat chest)? Or do you inhale more, retaining some breath, with more of a rounded, inflated chest? Or is your breathing balanced?

Type I breather (tendency toward exhalation)

With this kind of breathing, you are likely to run out of energy; you lack stamina. This type of breather is needy, even if the neediness is subtly expressed in the personality. Many times, this neediness is compensated for by special feats and brilliant accomplishments, masked by the consumption of stimulants, like nicotine and coffee. Still, this basic feeling forms your life.

A thorough change is attainable only through a change in the rhythm of the breath. The breath forms the basis of your life. The quality of your breath defines the quality of your actions and your experiences, the quality of your thoughts and moods.

Be aware that a thorough change in your breathing rhythm will lead to a drastic and far-reaching transformation of your feelings about life. New possibilities will manifest themselves, perhaps things that you have wished for but couldn't attain. Perspectives you have never thought existed will open themselves to you. But be aware that there might be resistance to doing the following exercises regularly because your organism is accustomed to a certain way of breathing, and all of your mental patterns and emotional habits depend on the way you are breathing now.

The goal of this exercise is to turn your breathing rhythm into its opposite. Breathe in deeply, hold your breath, then breathe out short and shallow, and fill your chest anew with oxygen. Keep repeating this for at least a quarter of an hour. For the first few days, it is recommended that you keep the following rhythm: four beats while inhaling, four beats holding your breath, and two beats while exhaling. After this, you can double the sequence: eight beats while inhaling, eight holding your breath, and four beats while exhaling.

You can do this exercise while listening to music, driving the car, washing dishes, reading the newspaper, talking, dancing, or playing with children. But if you have trouble doing the exercise for 15 minutes while occupied with other things, then do it in your room where you will not be interrupted.

What is important is the regularity with which you do this. Do the exercise every day for a month and keep a journal about it. Then take stock of what has happened in the meantime. If you have the feeling that it helps you to develop new parts of yourself, do it for three months.

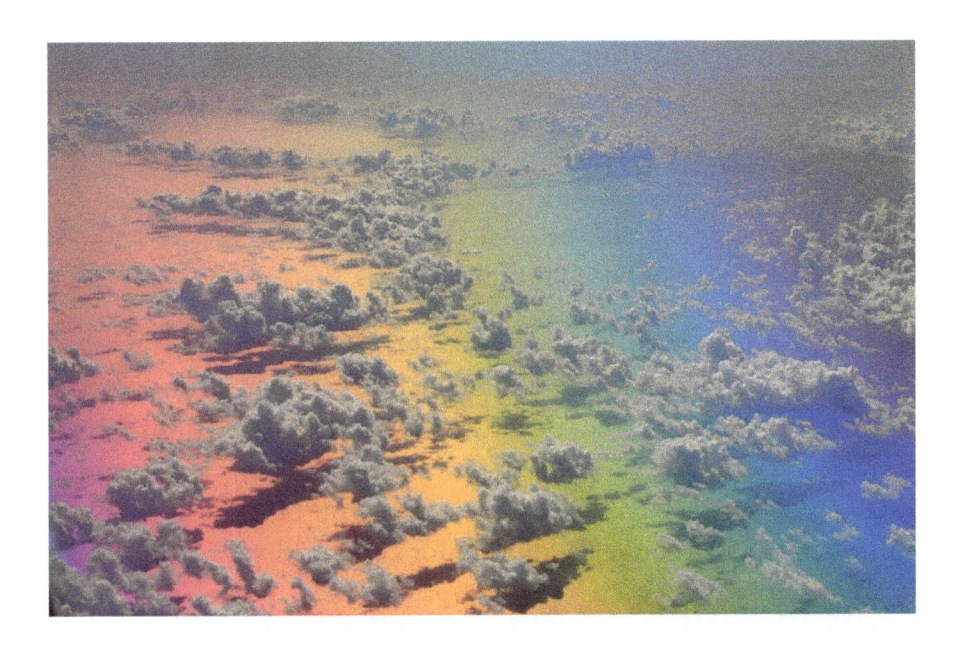

Type II breather (tendency toward inhalation)

You strut with an inflated chest through the world and like to make a show of your power. You hold on tightly to what you have: your image. It is difficult for you to let go of this image and show your weaknesses. You have learned that you are loved and admired when you are strong. Due to this, you take on a rather stiff and rigid attitude and cannot easily give way or yield. Your life has a somewhat static quality, and perhaps you have wondered why, with all the power you have and all the admiration you receive, you still are not completely satisfied.

If a few of these characteristics are on the mark, try the following exercise: exhale intensely, pause before the next inhalation, take a short and shallow breath, exhale intensely, and so on. For the first few days, follow this rhythm: four beats while exhaling, pause for four beats, and two beats while inhaling. Later you can double the rhythm: eight beats while exhaling, pause for eight beats, and four beats while inhaling. The rules for the last exercise apply to this one.

Appreciating grief

This is a difficult exercise because the ability to grieve and let go is not very well developed in our culture.

At the next opportunity, take time to grieve. It could be at the loss of a relative or a friend, or it could be a bad fight with your partner in which you weren't able to come to an agreement. Withdraw and feel your grief; don't suppress it. In case you don't have a reason to grieve, put yourself in a situation where you become sad: Spend some time in an orphanage or a senior care facility.

Concentrating on what is important

Write letters to people who mean a lot to you or who have meant a lot to you. Express your feelings and thoughts, above all the conflicts and problems that you have kept to yourself. Try to clear up misunderstandings and concentrate on what is important.

Exercises for the Lung and Large Intestine Meridians

Strengthening the Metal-Yin

The Lung posture

This posture embodies the essence of Lung energy — optimism, confidence, and trust in the future.

Take this posture when you feel discouraged and downcast, or when self-doubt blocks you from taking action. While taking this posture, visualize the Lung Meridian. It flows from the shoulder to the thumb. Intensify the energy flow in your imagination with every exhalation.

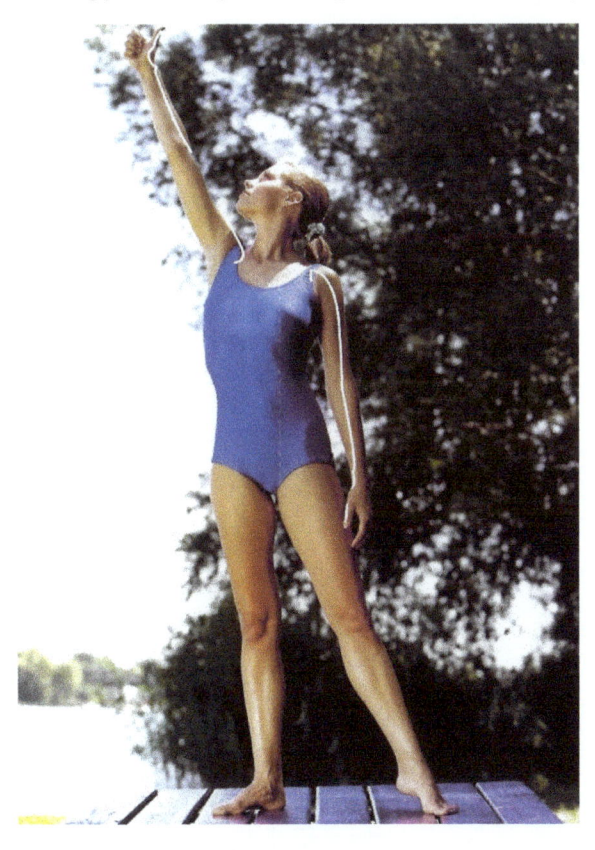

Activating the Lung Meridian

1. Stand with your feet parallel and three feet apart, shoulders relaxed, arms hanging down loosely. Your knees should be slightly bent.

2. Stretch your arms out in front of you to the height of your shoulders with your palms facing the ground.

3. While breathing in, swing your arms swiftly as far as possible to the left. Let your hips and your upper body follow. Your head should follow the movement of your upper body. Imagine that you are hurling something powerfully to the left. Let the motion take you as far as possible behind you in order to attain the greatest extension of the spine and long back muscles. Keep your arms parallel.

4. While breathing out, bring your arms back in front of you to the middle.

5. While breathing in, swing your arms as far as possible to the right (as above), and while breathing out, back to the middle.

6. Do this exercise for approximately five minutes.

Metal • 99

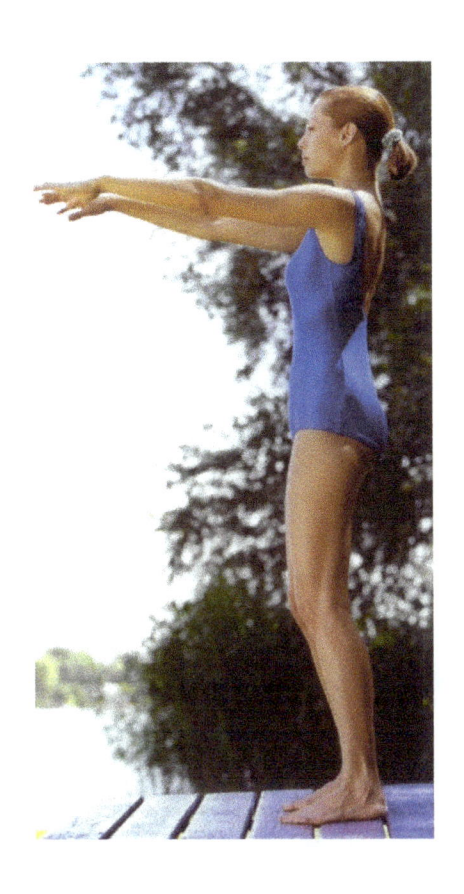

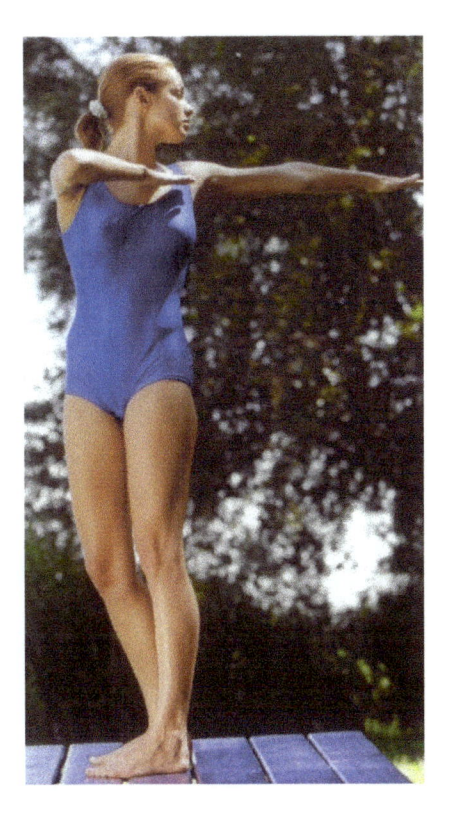

Strengthening the Metal-Yáng

The Large Intestine posture

This posture speaks for itself. The intellectual function of the Large Intestine is reflection and the elimination of mental waste: letting go of wishes, expectations, and ideas.

Take this posture when you have the feeling that you have gotten stuck on an idea or when you don't know how to move on.

The energy flows in the Large Intestine Meridian from the index finger, along the outside of the arm and over the shoulder and neck, to a point just next to the nostril. Visualize the Flow, white in color, with every inhalation.

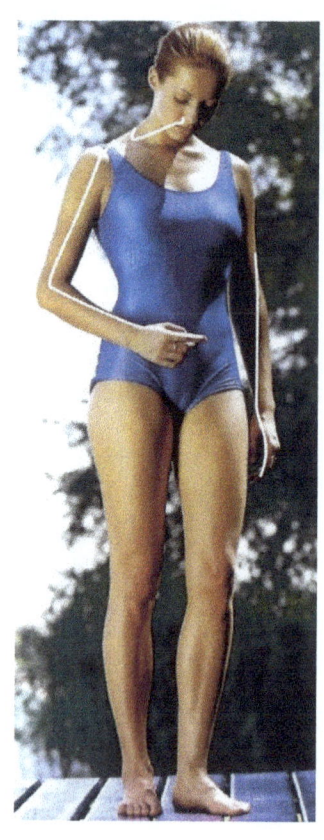

Activating the Large Intestine Meridian

1. In a standing position, cross your arms over your chest so that the palms of your hands are facing your shoulders.

2. This exercise is called "tightening the bow." While inhaling, straighten and stretch your left arm out to the side (the left hand is holding the bow) and "tighten the string" with your right hand in front of your chest. Your face should be turned to the left, the first finger of your left hand stretched out so that you can see your fingernail. Let the tension build. Through this tension, the Large Intestine Meridian is stimulated.

3. While exhaling, release the arrow from the bow and cross your arms over your chest, as in the beginning of the exercise.

4. Repeat the movements on the right side.

5. Do this exercise for one minute.

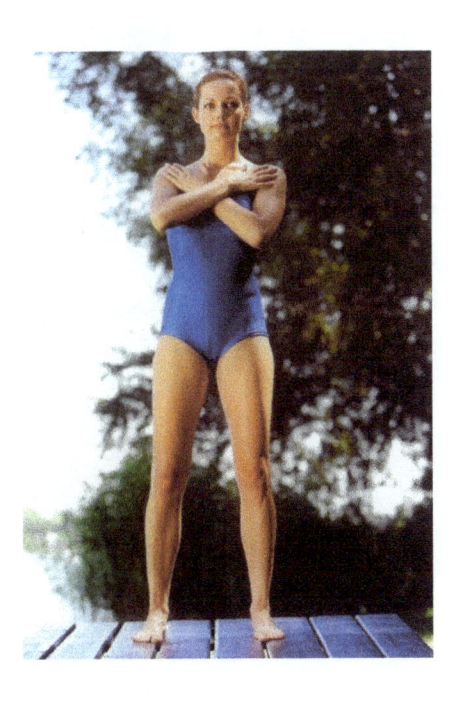

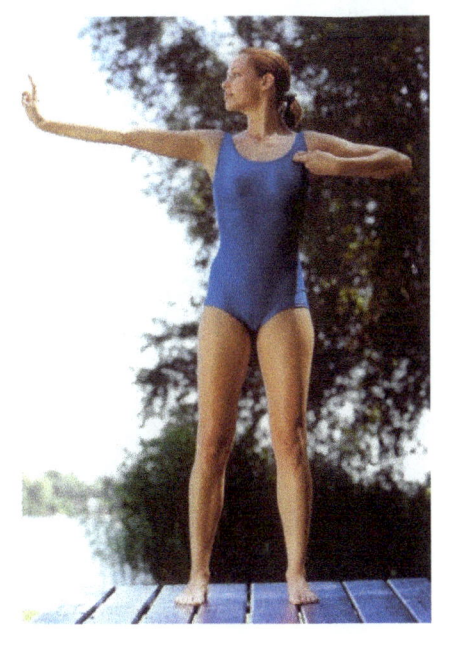

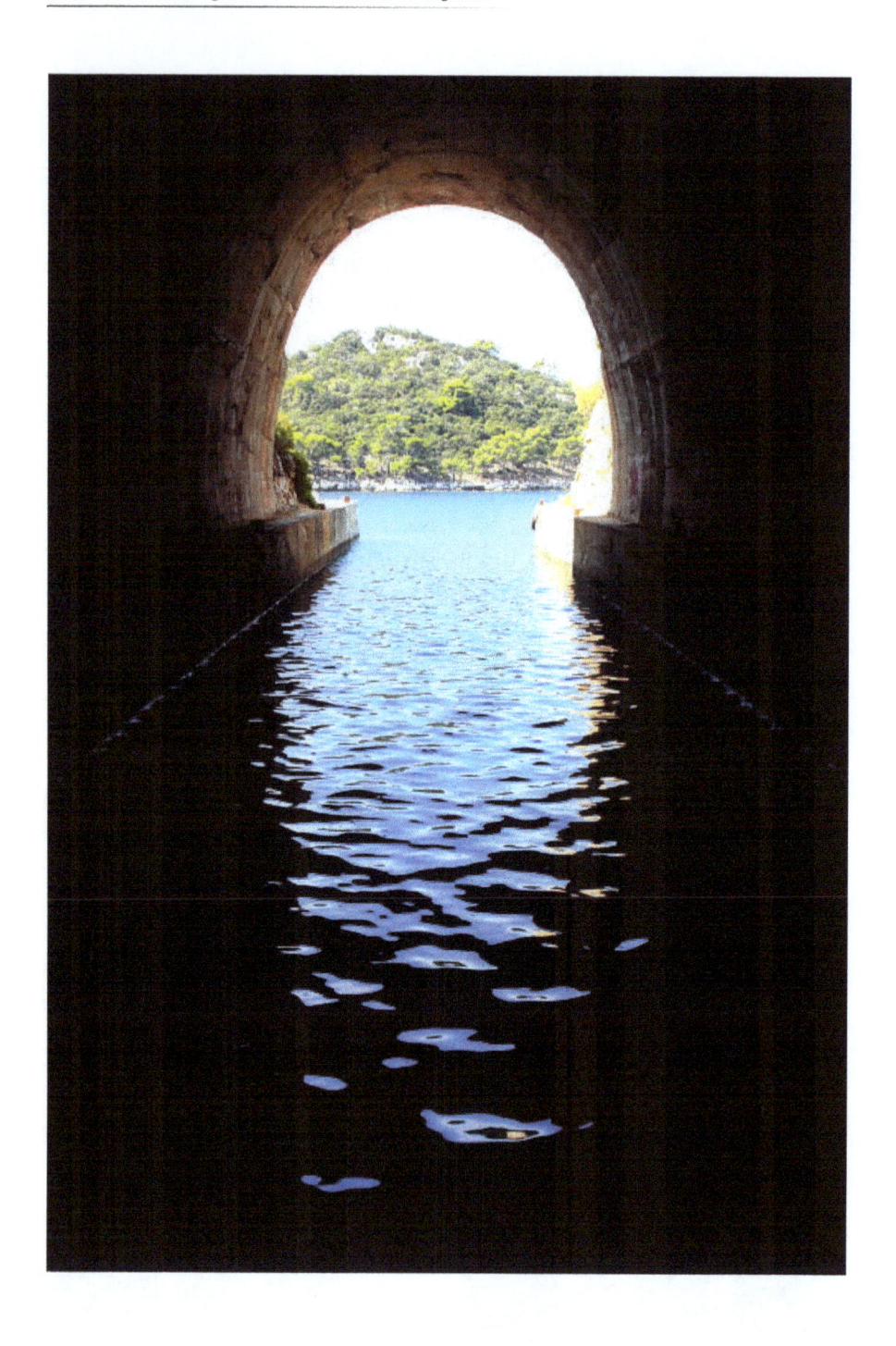

Water 水

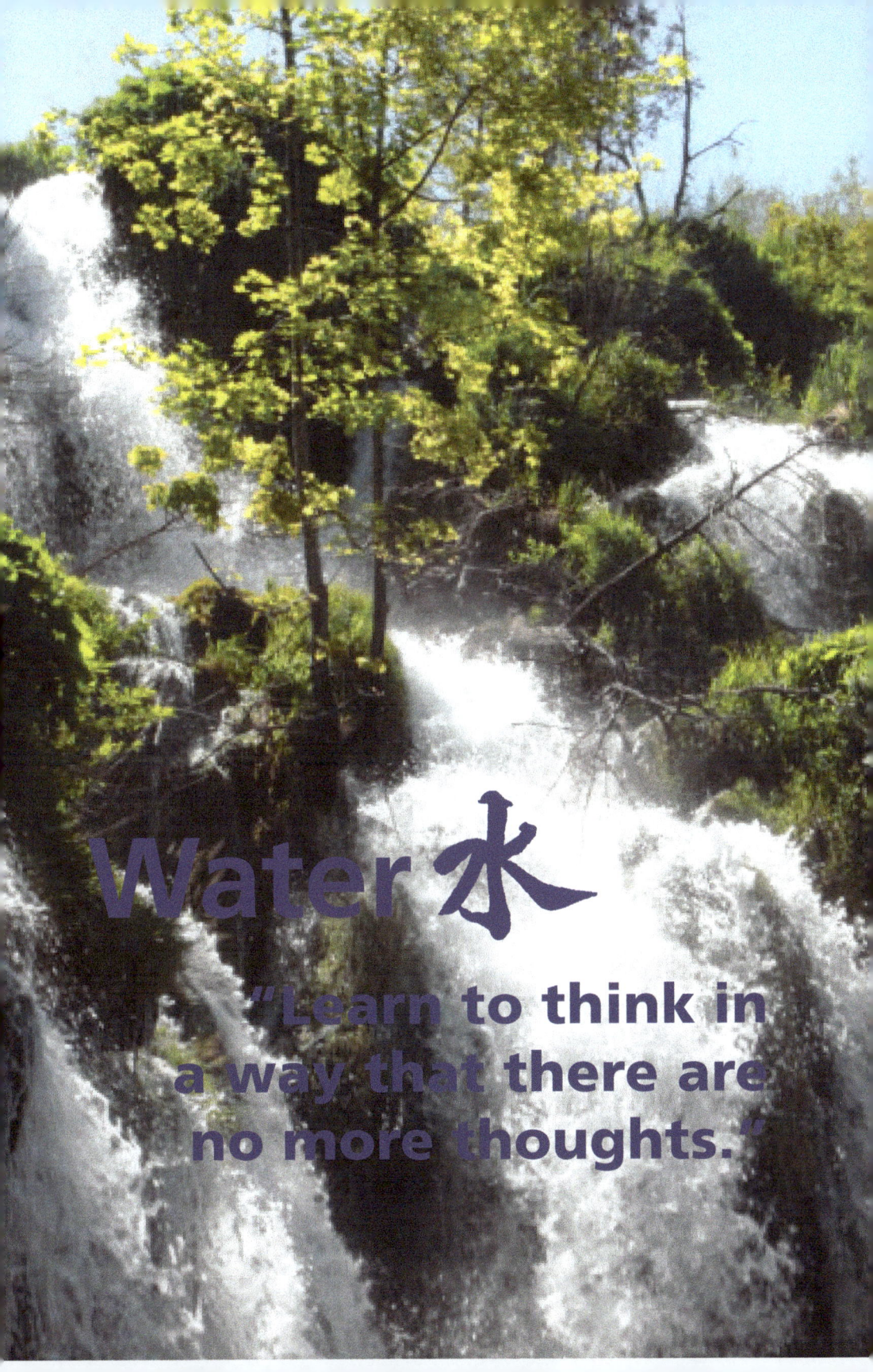

"Learn to think in a way that there are no more thoughts."

The Element Water

The season of Water is winter, the season of short days and long nights. The land lies under a blanket of snow, and the sun does not warm. Life has withdrawn into the ground; the power of life lies dormant in the seeds. Winter is the period between death and rebirth.

Water was called the "old Yin," the cold darkness. Its feeling is fear — the existential fear associated with survival. Its direction is north, its color black, and its time night. The Yin organ of Water are the Kidneys, its Yáng organ is the Bladder, and its tissue are the bones.

The character of Water is a sinking below; its energy is a vertical flow to the center of the earth. While the energy of Fire is directed above, toward the sky, Water pulls us into the depths. It acts on the physical body like the force of gravity and leads the soul and life back to its origin, to a deep consciousness, to the central core. The river picks up the stream and leads it back to the sea.

The nature of Water manifests itself in the image of the seed; compressed in a tiny space lies the potential for a large tree, the potential for a divergent development and unfolding. The seed is the essence of the tree. In the Chinese tradition, this essence was designated as the Ancestral Energy. The Kidneys are its guardian. The Ancestral Energy is the quality and quantity of varied energies that one inherits from one's parents and ancestors. The term "Ancestral Energy" is similar to our term "genetic code," whose 64 possible combinations are also found as symbols in the 64 Hexagrams of the *I Ching*. The Kidney is looked upon as the storage space for the Ancestral Energy, and also as a reservoir for different materials and fine energies, which, through the intake and processing of food, get into our organism and cannot be used immediately in life processes. It is said in the *Nei Ching*: "The Kidneys receive the essence of Zàng and Fu (organs) and store them."

A few names of points on the Bladder and Kidney Meridians reveal the effect that these points have on the energy storer: Bladder 24, "Conducts the Qì to the Sea of Energy"; Bladder 26, "Conducts the Qì to the Sea of Ancestral Energy"; Kidney 1, "Bubbling Spring"; Kidney 6, "Toward the Sea"; Kidney 13, "Nest of Life Force"; and, a point closely associated with the Kidney and Bladder, Governor 4, called Mìng Mén, "Gate of Life."

The traditional Chinese view — that the Kidneys house the genetic constitution — does not contradict the fact that every cell in the organism contains DNA and RNA because the Kidneys, like any other organ, are seen as a field of force that extends throughout the body. The anatomical Kidneys, as well as the bones and the ears, are the places in the body where the "Kidney Energy Field" condenses and materializes. The force of Water, however, like the energy of the other elements, affects every tissue and every cell. On a cellular level, the "Kidney Energy Field" is seen in connection with the chromosomes, the carriers of the genetic constitution. One could say that the wide variety of structures, forms, and processes found in human, animal, and plant organisms is a result of overlapping and constantly interacting energy fields. In ancient China, the constantly moving fields of forces were called the Elements.

The force of Water is present in various forms in the organism. Water is a flowing building block of the body; it constitutes 65% of the body weight and acts as a solvent and a lubricant. In the Chinese tradition, the Kidneys were labeled the controller of the water supply. In farming communities in China, the controller of the water supply held a highly honored position. He regulated the distribution of water for the rice fields in the different municipalities. The constant purification of the organism through water is made possible by the Kidneys and is one of its most important functions. The flow of water through the body has nothing to do with nourishment; that is the job of the Stomach and Pancreas. Water also doesn't provide the body with life energy, that job is taken care of by the Lungs.

Water flows without color and without form. Throughout the body, it picks up waste products, prevents stagnation, and makes movement, freshness, and "fluidity" of the body possible. There is no bodily function, no life process, that can be carried out without water. The inner secretions require water, and water is needed in the course of the digestive process, wherein food is taken in and transformed into a pulp (this is where the epithet, "Kidneys, Passage to the Stomach," comes from). Water is also needed to moisten the body orifices of eyes, mouth, nose, ears, sexual organs, and anus. And it is necessary for the control of body temperature through perspiration and the maintenance of the joint and muscle fluids.

The taste assigned to Water is salty. Salt regulates the amount of water retained by the body. The saltwater of the sea was the place of origin for all life on this planet, and the human body still has an internal sea-water environment, only slightly modified. The physiological mixture of the various salts in the blood and in the tissue fluids is, even after a million years, still similar to the composition of sea water. A surplus of salt in the organism leads to an accumulation of fluid in the tissues and therefore to swelling, edema, and weight gain.

Water rules the bones and, together with the Spleen, the Bone Marrow. The Kidneys are responsible for maintaining the right composition of salts and minerals in the blood; this is important for the building of the bones as well as for many other life processes. Without the right amount of salts and minerals in the body, the nerves cannot function, the muscles cannot move, and the Heart cannot beat. Therefore, it becomes clear why the Chinese find the Kidneys as important as the Heart: The Kidneys ensure the maintenance of the inner environment, the basis of life.

The conduction of nerve impulses especially depends on exact ion concentrations. Since the Kidneys are responsible for maintaining the right balance of ions in the blood and, thus, in the whole body, there is a close connection between the functioning of the Kidneys and the nervous system. This might be why the Chinese assigned the Brain and spinal cord to the Water element; in ancient Chinese texts, the Brain is called the "Sea of Marrow."

I assume that, 2,000 years ago, the Chinese did not know about ion concentrations and neurological processes as we do today. They had a different approach to reality. They thought more in analogies, and their logical processes were more influenced by intuitive insights. Since they did not have the scientific tools that we have today, they had to rely on holistic thinking and insight. Thus, I imagine that the Brain was called the "Sea of Marrow," not because of the scientifically provable connection between the functioning of the Kidneys and neurological processes but because the Brain in the skull looks very similar to the marrow in the bone. If you have ever observed brain surgery in a movie, you will know what I mean. I assume that they were calling the Brain "Sea of Marrow," first, because of a pictorial and also tangible analogy and, second, because they were contemplating the various organs, body tissues, sense organs, and meridians throughout many centuries, and so they had attained an intuitively based and empirically verified knowledge about the connections between the various organs and meridians.

In the context of the nervous system, a few more things can be said about the relationship between Water and Fire. Life evolved in the sea, and the Water element is the base of our life, of our will to survive, of our vitality and sexual drive. The simple life forms are assigned to the Water element: A one-celled organism has no blood circulation and no heart; it is composed of a cell membrane, salt water, genetic material, and simple cell organs. In comparison to this, Fire, along with Metal and Earth, allows a higher order of things to come into being. This is why the material substance of the nervous system is assigned to Water, but the more complex phenomena of the transmission of stimuli and the coordination of electrical impulses in the nervous system are attributed to Fire. Water is the base, Fire is the top.

In the Chinese tradition, all of the hormones and glands are associated with the Water element. The ancient texts distinguish Yin-Kidney and Yáng-Kidney. The Yin-Kidney is also called the Water-Kidney, and the Yáng-Kidney the Fire-Kidney.

The Water-Kidney filters the blood and produces urine. On the physical level, it corresponds to the Kidney with all its various functions as we know it in Western medicine. The Fire-Kidney corresponds to the endocrine system: the Adrenal Glands, the sex glands, the islets of Langerhans in the Pancreas, the thyroid and thymus, and, finally, the pituitary gland.

The concept of the Water-Kidney and Fire-Kidney also indicates the nature of the elemental spirit of Water, the Zhì. Zhì is our willpower, our will to survive, and our sexual drive. It represents the vitality with which a person masters life. Zhì can unfold when the organism is flowing freely, fresh and clean inside, and when the hormones are working so well together that the metabolic processes are well tuned. Then a bubbly, fiery power and vitality can develop. This power manifests itself in supple body movements, flexible joints, sexual potency, strong bones and healthy teeth, a silky shine to the hair, good hearing, a tremendous urge for action and activity, and a healthy ability to adjust to the demands of circumstances. The balance of the element Water is dependent upon the relationship between the Yin-Kidney and the Yáng-Kidney. When the Fire-Kidney is weak or when there is surplus energy in the Yin-Kidney in contrast to the Yáng-Kidney, the will to live, vitality, and sexual drive decrease. The results may be a general weakness, impotence, frigidity, and paralyzing fear.

When the energy of the Yáng-Kidney is dominant, one often finds a person who is constantly in a hurry or a person with rigid behavior and body movements. This rigidity and stiffness manifests itself, above all, in the lower back, the ilio-sacral joints, and the backs of the legs along the course of the Bladder Meridian. The symptoms of this rigidity are a hollow back, disk problems in the lumbar vertebrae, sciatica, lumbago, and bladder infections.

Other consequences of an imbalance in Water are kidney stones, kidney and urinary tract infections, bone diseases, loss of hair, some types of watery diarrhea, menstrual disorders, insomnia, and constantly cold legs and feet.

The Kidneys rule the ears and hearing. The balance of the fluid in the ear is crucial to the quality of our hearing. Our sense of balance — a function made possible by the right combination of fluid in the labyrinth of the ear — is also assigned to Water. Most illnesses concerning the ears — inflammation of the middle ear, buzzing in the ears, hearing difficulties, deafness, or dizziness — can be traced to a disturbance in the Water element.

The hormones are produced by the Adrenal Glands and their function explains the emotions and drives associated with Water. On the one hand, there are the androgens with their direct effect on the libido; on the other hand, there are adrenaline, noradrenaline, cortisol, and aldosterone, which regulate blood pressure and the balance of fluids in the body. A real or imagined danger that causes us to be afraid is the strongest stimulus that sets off the release of these hormones in the circulatory system. In China, fear is associated with the tremendous power of Water, which shows itself in floods set off by earthquakes and tidal waves triggered by typhoons. Fear is also associated with a Water deficiency, such as when the fields dry out and famine is imminent.

As with the other elements, there are emotions and feelings associated with the force of Water that express a balance or imbalance in this element. When one has all five senses together and balanced, it is natural to feel afraid in dangerous situations. We are afraid of something concrete; we recognize the danger in time and can take action to get away from what is threatening us. Fear ensures our biological survival. Through fear, we learn to respect life and its awesome power.

Compared to fear, anxiety and terror are more intense; they are emotional states in which the actual threat can no longer be properly assessed. Often, the threat is imaginary and illusory. Anxiety is a state in which either a threat cannot be judged correctly or the danger no longer exists. The word "anxiety" stems from the Latin word *angustia*, which can be translated as "narrowness, restriction, conciseness, difficulty, poverty, need, and trouble." Anxieties develop when we have isolated ourselves and are no longer in harmony with things and people around us. Being able to resonate with our environment is a characteristic of the Water element: to be soft, to surrender oneself, and to not put up any resistance. Serious disturbances in Water lead to panic attacks, paranoia, a persecution complex, fear of the dark, fear of an inner "black hole," and situations in which one becomes rigid, immovable, and paralyzed with fear.

The Water element harbors the deepest secrets of life. When we accept the power of Water, we become quiet inside and the surface of the lake becomes smooth. In this inner quiet, the world of dreams, the realms of sleep, and the unconscious slowly open up. Step by step, the way through the realm of death also becomes visible. Water is the element of the deepening of self and meditation. If one is at home in the depths, one can meet the storms on the surface calmly. With Water, more than with any other element, we come across that which has no name, the Dào.

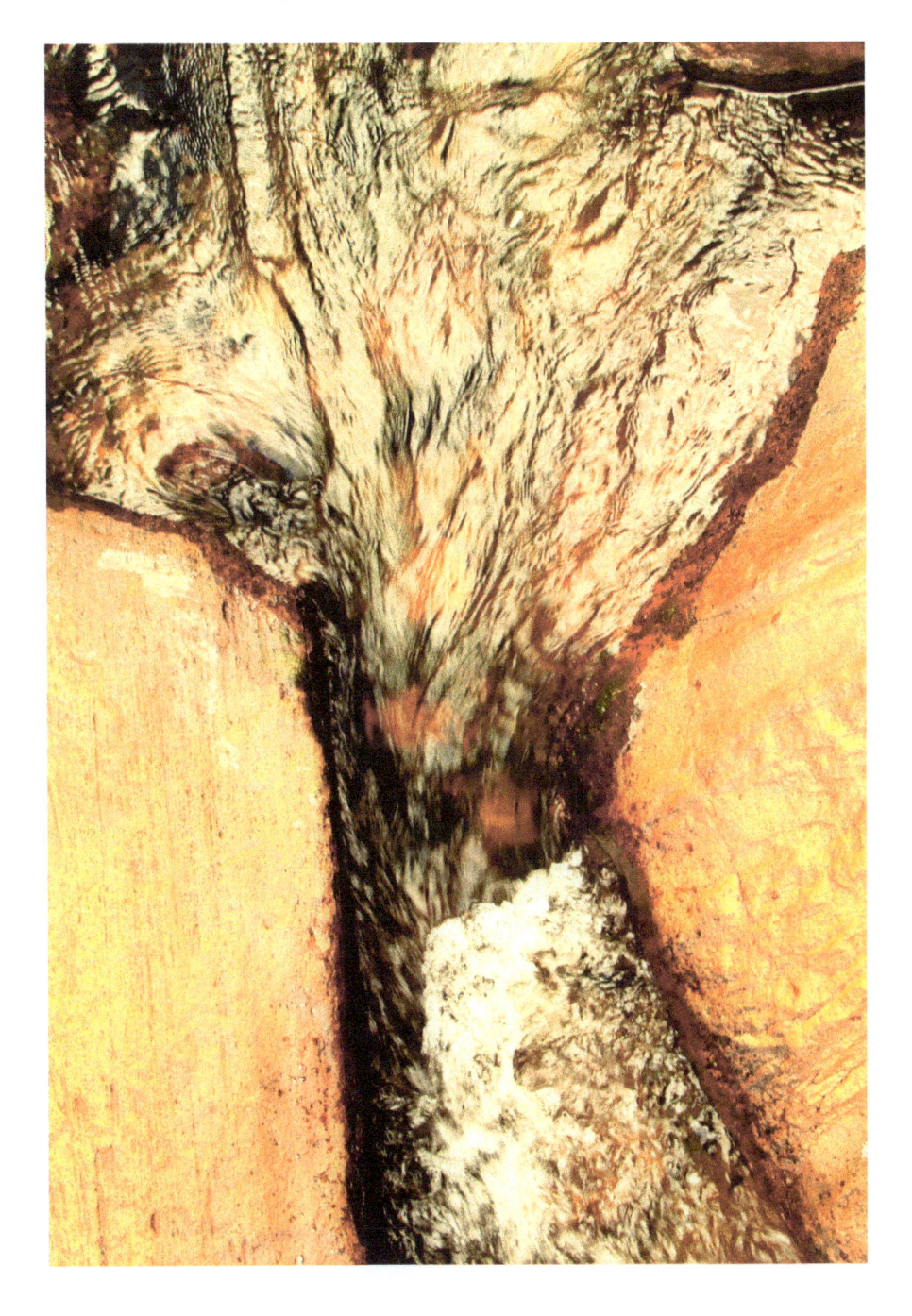

Mental and Physical Exercises to Get the Water Flowing

Clarifying questions

Proceed with the following questions as you have done previously.

- How do I feel in winter or when the weather is cold?
- Am I afraid of the dark?
- Do I have a strong will that helps me to overcome difficulties?
- Is my sex drive strong or weak?
- In what situations do I deeply relax?
- Can I delve into something to a point where everything else loses its meaning?
- Do I have a strong imagination or ability to fantasize?
- What am I afraid of?
- Do I have secrets?
- Do I hear well?
- Have I ever had inflammation of the middle ear or a buzzing in the ears that lasted for a long time?
- Is my hair healthy and strong?
- Do I have good dental health?
- Do I sometimes have discomfort or pain in the small of my back?
- Do I tend to get bladder infections?
- Have I ever had an illness of the Kidneys?
- Do I prefer savory food, or do I have an aversion to salt?

- Am I very ambitious, or not ambitious at all?
- What or whom do I respect or revere?
- What really amazed me last week?
- Have I ever thought about how I will die or how I would like to die?
- What is my attitude toward death?
- What do I think is the biggest secret in life?

Water exercises

Confronting your fear

Go into a dark room in the evening. Imagine a situation in which you were afraid, and recall it in your memory in detail. Let the situation appear worse to you than it was, and enter into your fear.

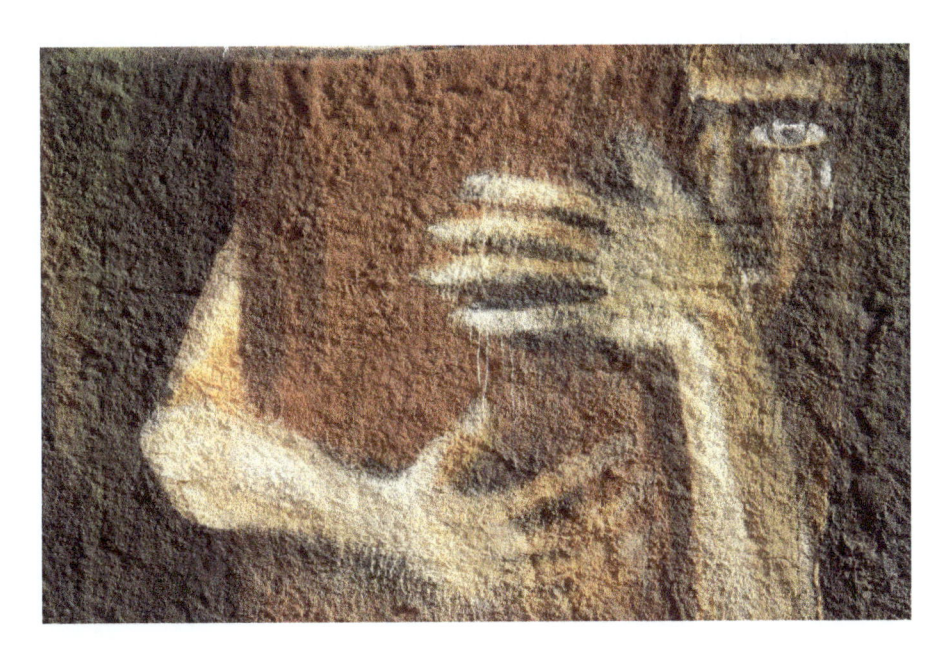

When you feel the fear deeply, focus your attention on your body. Where do you get cramped and tense? Do you hold your breath or take short, shallow breaths? Take a few deep, long breaths while you once again experience the fearful situation in your imagination. Keep breathing deeply until the fear lessens or completely disappears.

If you are a fearful person, do this exercise once a week for one to two months. It can help reduce your fears. Then, next time a dangerous situation arises, you will be able to react more calmly and defend yourself better.

Feeling the womb

Lie down on your bed in the afternoon or evening and close your eyes. Take approximately 15 minutes to journey into your past. Remember how you felt yesterday, a week ago, a year ago, three years ago, five years ago, and so on. Remember your puberty, your first years of school, your childhood. Imagine how you might have felt as an infant, at your birth, before your birth. If feelings or pictures from this time appear, let them come; do not try to interpret them or compare them to what you already know. Imagine that you are swimming in amniotic fluid. Then feel the slow, deep breaths of your mother as she sleeps, and how they rock you tenderly. Imagine this breath that surrounds you and is bigger than you, that rocks you and keeps you safe. And then let your own tiny breath become synchronized with this bigger breath. Simply listen to it; don't do anything else. The breath goes in. The breath goes out. The breath goes in. The breath goes out.

Listen for about 15 minutes to the breath in silence.

Latihan

This is a technique of the Tantra tradition. It releases the "flow of water" in us — the ability to be soft, to be yielding, to let things happen, to flow.

Go into a dark room in the evening. Wear comfortable clothes and take off your shoes and socks. Dance a fantasy dance for 15 minutes so that you become loose and relaxed.

Then stand in the middle of the room and don't move; don't do anything. Relax, but refrain from moving. After a few minutes, you will sense that your body begins to stir on its own. Let it move exactly as it wants to; don't interfere. Perhaps you will feel a twitch, or a small quiver may go through your body. A movement begins, is interrupted, and then continues. Follow the dynamic of your body.

After a while, you will feel charged. Whenever you turn off your arbitrary motor, deeper centers in the Brain take over the controls, and suppressed movements can come to the surface. Tension and blocks eventually release themselves under the influence of self-regulated centers, and the muscle tone changes. Energy is released.

Remain in this state for about 30 minutes. Then lie on your back and enjoy the relaxed feeling you have.

Exercises for the Bladder and Kidney Meridians

Strengthening the Water-Yáng

The Bladder posture

The function of the Bladder has to do with mental and physical relaxation, letting go of activity, and returning to a quiet state.

Take this posture when you have done strenuous work and would like to relax. Swing slowly from one side to the other and back again.

Then change the direction for a while. Let your upper body fall forward without making an effort to do so, then stand up again and arch backward to stretch your back and neck muscles. Do this several times.

With every repetition, let your body fall farther forward while visualizing the Bladder Meridian. It flows from the inner corner of the eye, over the head, down the back and the backs of the legs, along the outside of the foot to the small toe. Visualize it on your head and your back approximately two finger-widths to either side of the midline of your body.

Water • 117

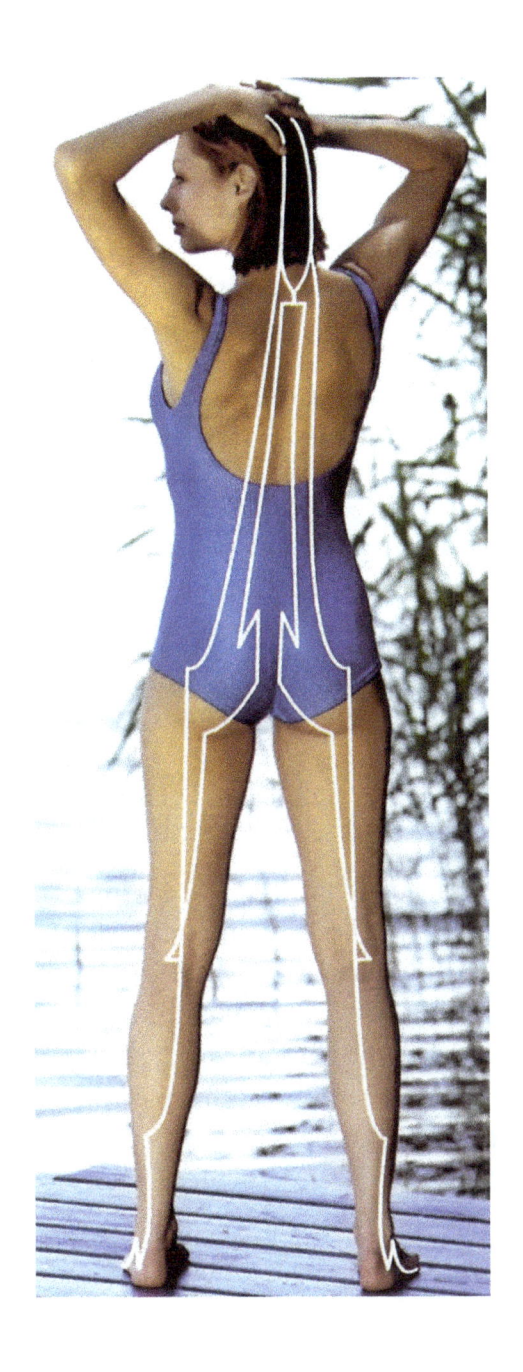

Activating the Bladder Meridian: The candle and the plow

1. The candle: Lie relaxed on your back, your arms at your sides.

2. Raise your legs to a vertical position.

3. Supporting your back with your hands, lift your lower torso so that it lies on the same vertical line as the legs. The weight of your body rests on your shoulders and neck. Each day, stay a bit longer in this posture, up to three minutes.

4. Then proceed slowly to the plow: keeping your legs straight, slowly bring them over your head until your toes are touching the ground. Hold your legs as straight as you can without feeling a painful tension. Relax and breathe into your abdomen. Remain in this position for up to three minutes.

5. Keeping your legs straight, raise them slowly back to a vertical position until you are in the candle posture again.

6. Lower your legs slowly until you are lying on your back. Take at least a minute to relax and enjoy the effects of this exercise. The candle and the plow are Hatha Yoga exercises that stretch and activate the Bladder Meridian. They loosen the spine, the cramped muscles in the neck and back, and the backs of the legs. They relieve the Heart by promoting blood flow in the veins and preventing edema in the legs and varicose veins.

Water • 119

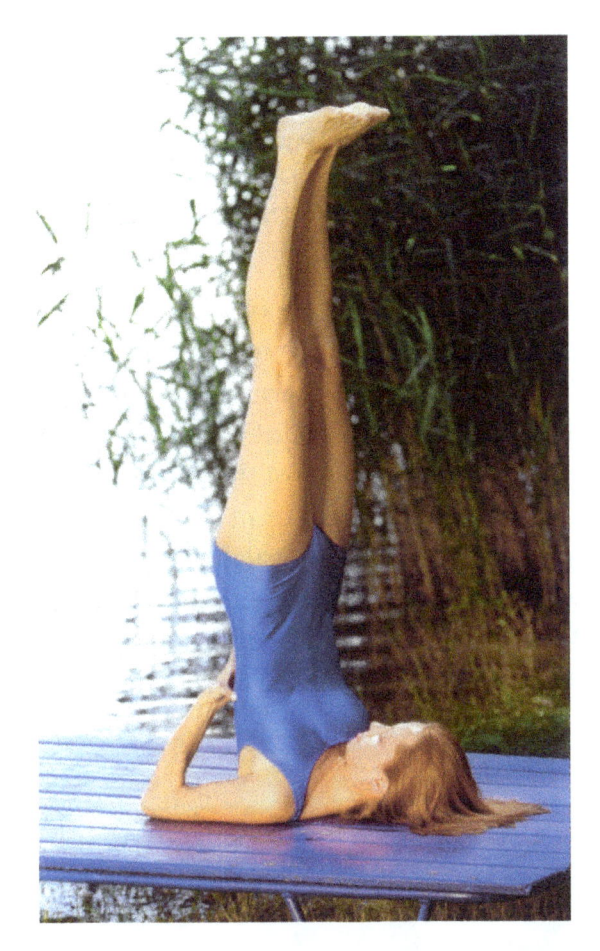

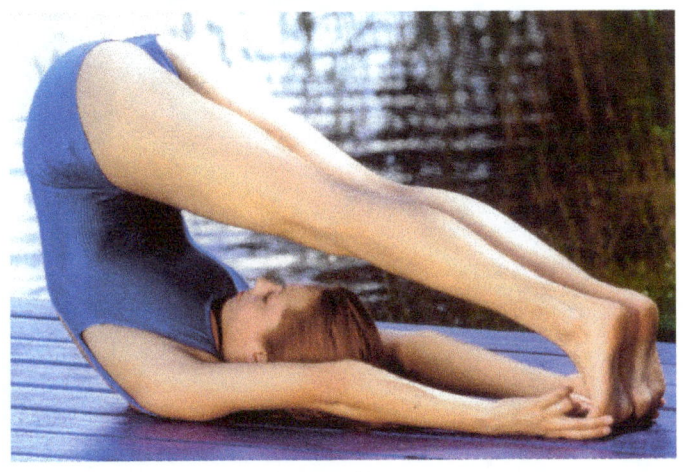

Strengthening the Water-Yin

The Kidney posture

This position depicts the essence of the Kidneys: trust, flow, regeneration, and quiescence.

The Kidney Meridian flows from the sole of the foot along the inside of the leg to the pelvic floor, and from there, it ascends along the spine to the lower back. From Mìng Mén (Governor 4), at the level of the second lumbar vertebra, it goes to the Kidneys and, along the Ureters, to the Bladder. It comes to the surface of the body again at the upper border of the pubic bone and ascends from there along the abdomen and the chest up to the collar bone. Visualize the Kidney Meridian in the bent leg while you breathe in (the energy flow is less intense in the straight leg). Take the mirror image of this posture for a while and visualize the Kidney Meridian on the other side.

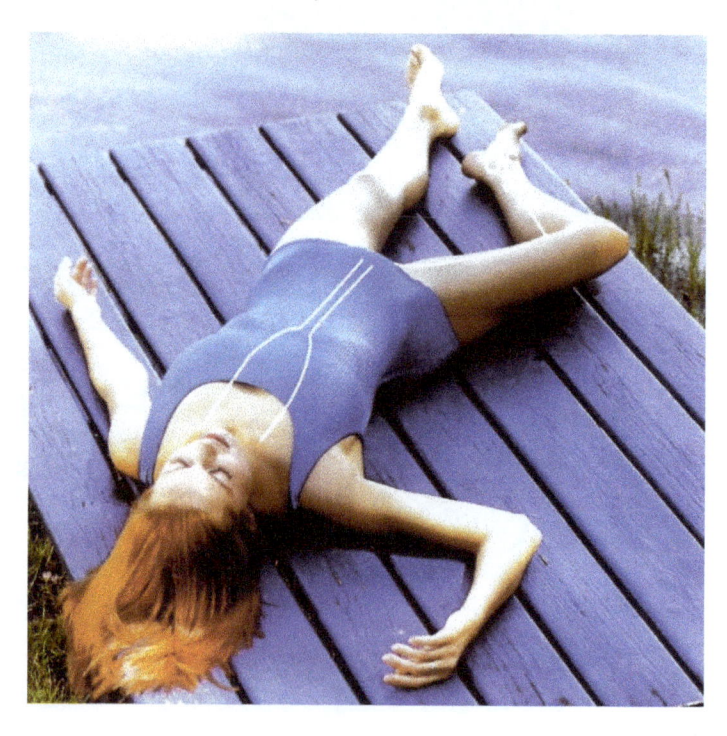

Activating the Kidney Meridian

1. Sit on the floor with your legs bent so that the soles of your feet are touching each other.

2. Hold your ankles and press the Kidney 6 point with your thumbs on both feet. This acupressure point lies one thumb-width under the tip of the inner ankle bone in the small indentation between the tendons.

3. Pull your feet as close to your pelvis as possible.

4. When you inhale, sit up and stretch your spine. When you exhale, bend your upper body, bringing your forehead as close to your toes as possible.

5. Do this exercise for a minute. Breathe deeply and regularly.

6. When you are finished, sit up straight with your legs crossed and close your eyes. When you exhale, say the mantra "Zhì" to yourself for 1–3 minutes.

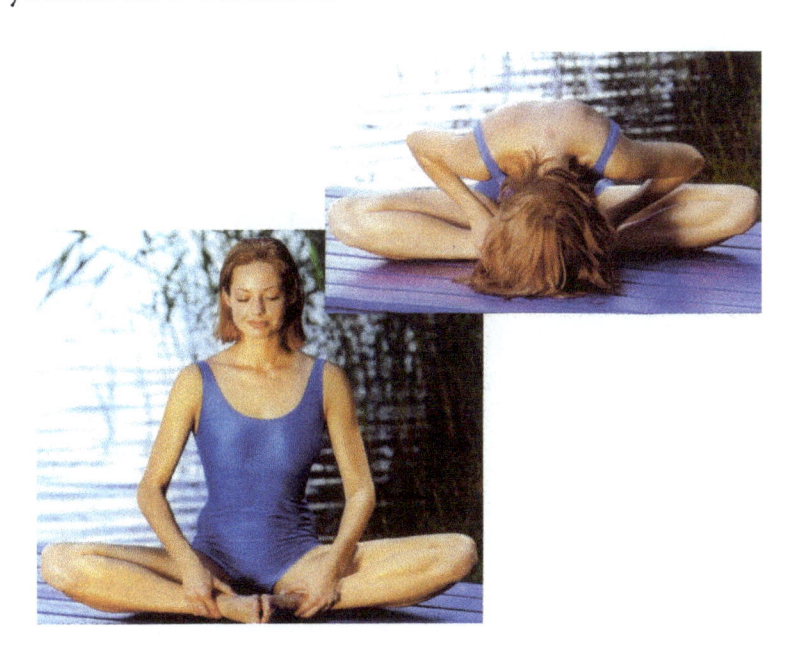

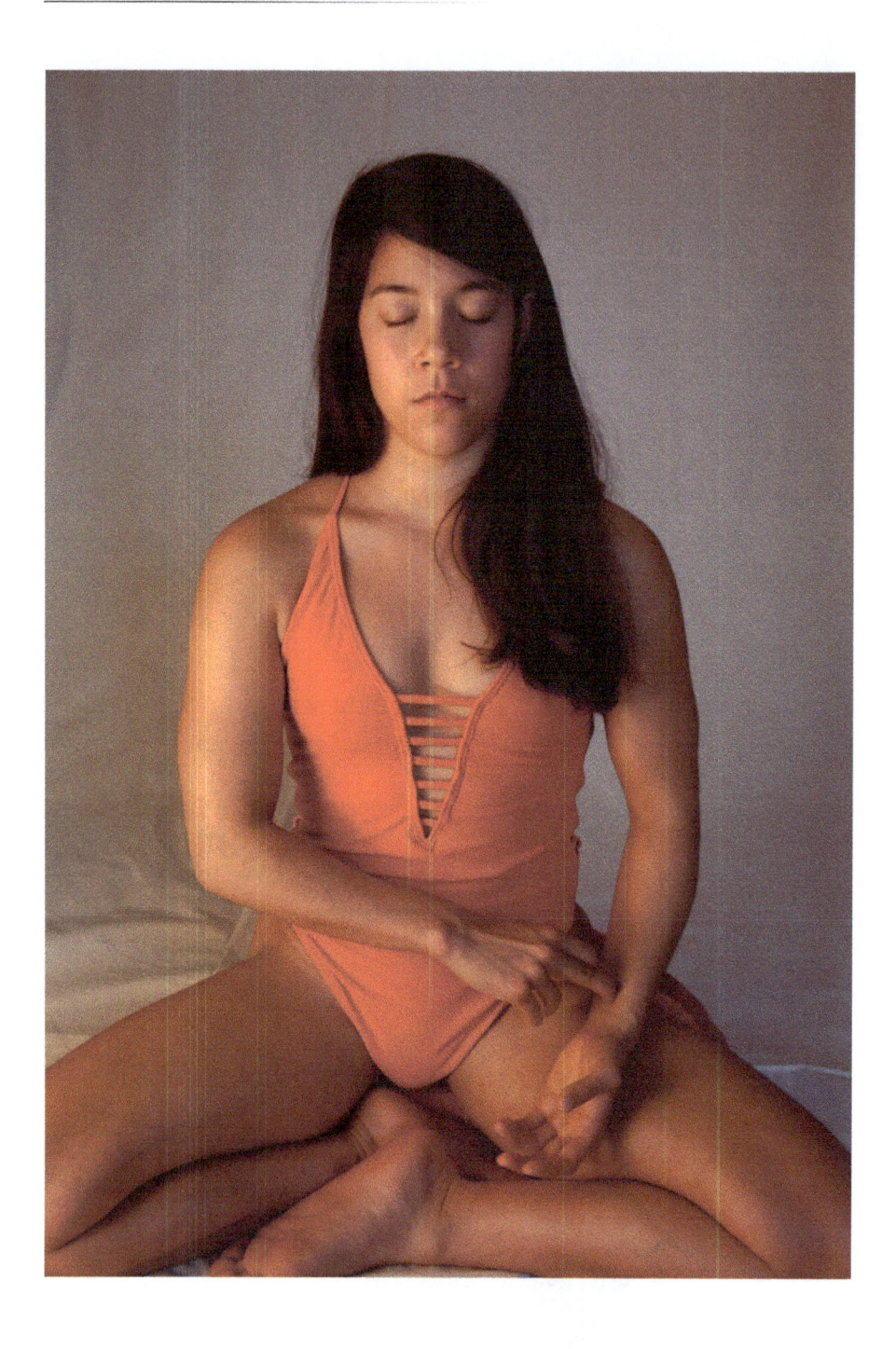

The Four Cycles

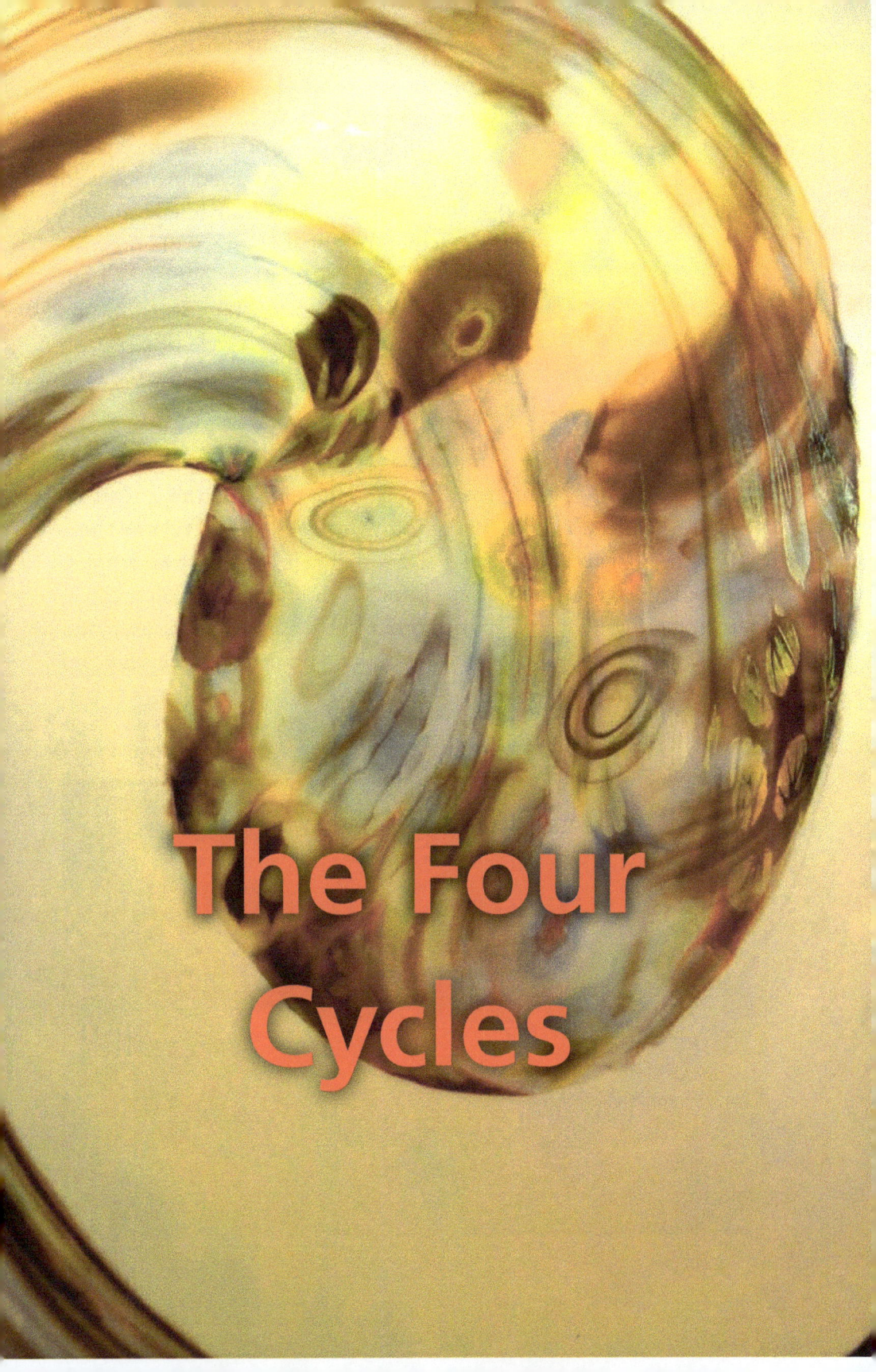

The Chinese placed a great deal of importance on the harmony and balance of the forces and energies. For the observed processes in nature and the cosmos, the characteristics of the individual elements play less of a role than their actual interplay. In every life process, the elements balance each other, create each other, and block each other. The Chinese tradition recognizes four laws governing the relationship of the elements to each other: the Cycle of Creation (Shéng), the Cycle of Checking-Up and Control (Ko), the Cycle of Rebellion, and the Cycle of Withdrawal.

These four cycles describe the phases of growth and the physiological interplay of the organs. They describe the path and the spreading of complaints and diseases from one element to another, from one organ to another. The four cycles make the complex combinations that form the basis for the individual clinical pictures understandable. If one applies them to the emotional and mental levels, one gets an overview of the dialectic between feelings and mental attitudes.

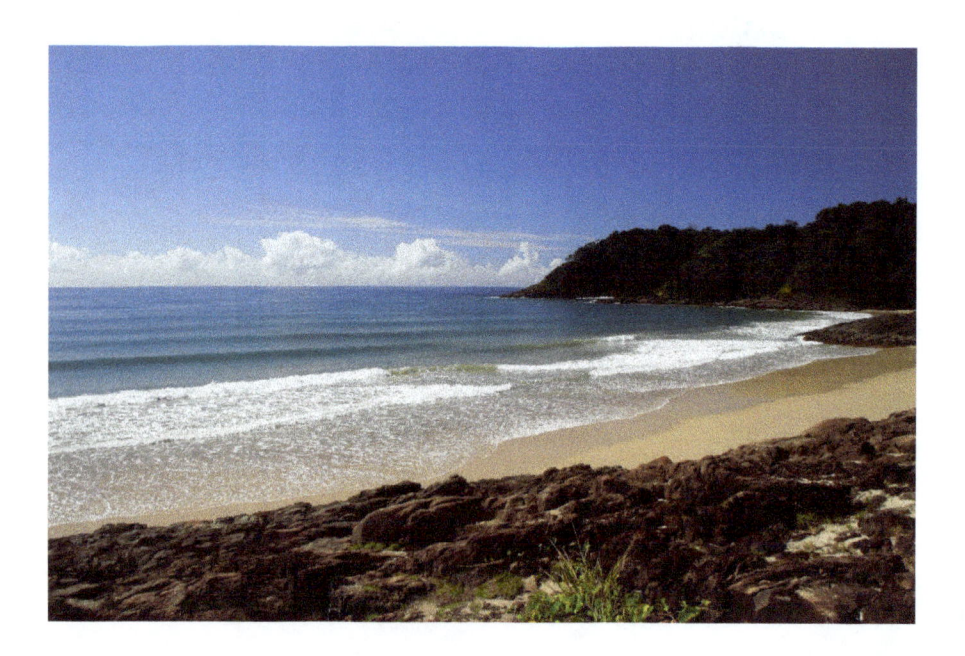

The cycles also describe the personality structures as well as the connection between personality and illness. They are a basic instrument of traditional Chinese diagnosis and therapy. The four cycles show how the elements are connected to each other, and how everything that happens has an effect on everything else.

The Shéng Cycle or the Law of Mother and Child

This cycle describes the transition from one element to the next, from one phase to the next. Wood transforms into Fire, Fire into Earth, Earth into Metal, Metal into Water, and Water back into Wood. In Chinese texts, the changes are shown in the following way: You use wood to make fire; when the fire has burned, it becomes ashes, it becomes earth; in the depths of the earth, metals and minerals are compressed and created; water condenses on metal, or out of heaven, the kingdom of metal, comes the rain; water nourishes the plants so they can grow, hence, water creates wood; when a lot of wood is piled up, then the fire will burn brighter and longer; the burning of fields creates new, fertile earth. The manifestation of energy of every element is dependent upon the nourishment it gets from the element before it in the cycle; therefore, this cycle is also called the Cycle of Nourishment.

Nourishment and building are attributed to the Yin, so the Shéng cycle is particularly effective in the Yin organs. The Liver (Wood Yin) nourishes the Heart, the Heart (Fire Yin) nourishes the Spleen, the Spleen (Earth Yin) nourishes the Lungs, the Lungs (Metal Yin) nourish the Kidneys, the Kidneys (Water Yin) nourish the Liver, and so on.

It is difficult to translate the principles described here into terms understood in Western physiology. The Shéng cycle describes the transformation of dynamic powers and energies that have reflections

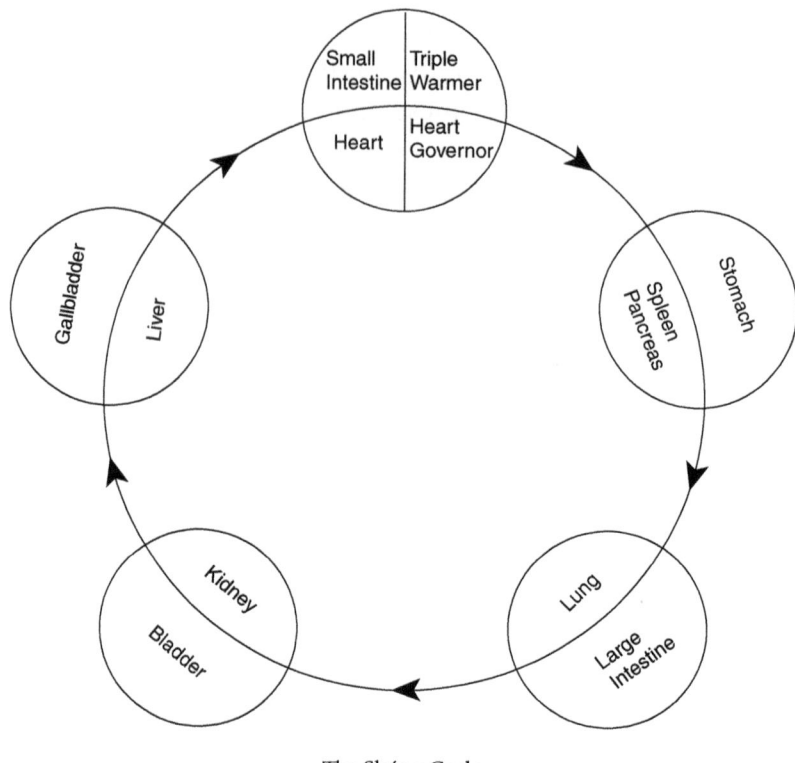

The Shéng Cycle

on the organic and mental levels. It is not possible to measure the energies, but one can recognize their effects.

For example, in the practice of Chinese medicine, the Kidneys are strengthened through the Lung energy. This combination is often found in illnesses. If the first imbalances and illnesses in childhood are in Metal and are manifested in chronic colds, whooping cough, pneumonia, or diarrhea, then, in the next period of growth, one is likely to find imbalances in Water, manifested in middle-ear infections, buzzing in the ears, or tooth decay. In this case, Water and its organs and tissues were undernourished for years because Metal was weak.

The Shéng cycle portrays a closed circle. If the circle is broken at any point and one element is unable to nourish the next, the result is "malnourishment." The Chinese call this, relative to the previous element, the "child." The nourishing element is the "mother." The child of one element is the mother of the next, and so on, until the circle is completed. Therefore, this cycle is called the Law of Mother and Child. The strength of an element is dependent on proper nourishment from the mother. One can observe this mother–child relationship in every area: biological, emotional, and mental. Undernourishment is important for diagnosis, but there are also diseases caused by overfeeding.

As clear as these laws may appear in an individual case, it is difficult to describe them abstractly. On an emotional level, one can best understand the transition of the feelings from one element to the next when one looks at the course of the year with its different seasons and the basic feelings that are associated with them. Spring is the time for new plans; new projects are started. People are more extroverted; they meet new people and fall in love anew. As the whole emotional spectrum of Wood is intensified during spring, some people may experience increased impatience and irritability on one hand if the Wood element is strong, and deep depression on the other hand if the Wood element is weak. The blooming of summer grows out of this new beginning in spring — the joy of succeeding, celebrating, and dancing. A person may feel relieved and conciliatory after a sudden release of anger; one has expressed oneself, stated one's opinion, and not stood in one's own way. The experience shows that people who never become angry rarely experience a real, pulsating joy. One can readily observe the transition from Wood to Fire in children. One minute they are hopping mad, insulting each other, arguing or fighting with each other, and the next minute they are best friends again and play as if there had never been anything wrong.

After a time of joy, we often linger in its wake and yearn to return to it. We become quieter, more reflective, maybe even melancholic. We rave about romance and experiences from the past. These are all moods of the element Earth. Empathy and sympathy can arise out of fully felt joy — a deep understanding and bonding with someone you love and with whom you have shared happiness. Out of the sympathy that has arisen from a shared high or peak experience, constructive criticism becomes possible — yet another characteristic of the element Earth.

Melancholy can result in sadness; empathy can lead to insight about whether and when it would be a good time to leave another person. A person who can feel the needs of another will know when it is time to go. Such a person will also know the right time to be alone and to draw within, not clinging to the other person, as is common with a person who has an overly strong Earth with a disturbed transition into Metal. A person who experiences a flowing transition from Earth to Metal is able to let go of the past, sever past bonds, and give up old identities. The essence of past experiences will be kept, and those that are not important will be released. Maturity will develop through grieving and letting go. If the transition from Metal to Water is incomplete, then the person will be afraid of being alone. Aloneness will be seen as loneliness and a yearning to bond with others. Behind the fear of loneliness is almost always the fear of being confronted with oneself and one's own unconscious. This is so because, in being alone, we experience through our own power who we really are. The ability assigned to the Metal element of letting go and taking leave of something or someone is necessary in order to arrive at the stillness of the Water and to become silent.

Out of the silence grows a new beginning. This is the transition from Water to Wood. On an emotional level, we experience this transition as a sudden change from fear to aggression. A person who is cornered and feels threatened may, out of fear, suddenly attack or feel paralyzed. The former shows a healthy transition from Water to Wood. One can see this especially clearly in animals and children. With inhibited people who were raised to be well behaved and to hold themselves back, the paralyzing form of fear dominates. One cannot imagine a way out or how to successfully prevail. The transition from Water to Wood is unbalanced. Plants cannot grow in salt water.

The Ko Cycle or the Law of Grandmother and Grandchild

The cycle of creation and building has, as its natural polarity, breakdown and destruction of outlived structures. Everything that grows has its natural limits beyond which the growth is no longer useful. If these limits are exceeded, an imbalance in the elements results, causing rampant growth, hypertrophy, and finally cancer.

Just as every element has a mother who nourishes it, every element also has a grandmother who is responsible for its upbringing and its proper growth. In ancient China, as in many other cultures, the grandparents had the job of recognizing the proper vocation for their grandchildren and furthering this by taking care of the training. They were the real authorities in the upbringing; they passed on the experience of generations, mostly in the form of narration or stories. They made the decisions concerning career and marriage. The parents, in contrast, took care of the material side of life; they worked in the fields and supported the family.

It is characteristic of our culture that the function of the grandparents, especially in cities, has become almost meaningless. The education and development of children are put in the hands of anonymous public schools, where a lot of information is given, but very little real knowledge is conveyed about one's destiny and the meaning of life. What remains is the function of the parents, who take care of supporting the family materially.

It was the responsibility of grandparents to give their grandchildren the direction and support necessary for their development. If the grandparents were too strict and their methods too authoritarian, the grandchildren did not develop independence in actions, thoughts, and feelings. If they let their grandchildren get away with too much and did not reprimand them enough, the grandchildren became too high-handed, arrogant, and incapable of being subordinate later in life.

The diagram of the Ko cycle shows a five-pointed star. In the mystical traditions of the Western world, this symbol is known as a

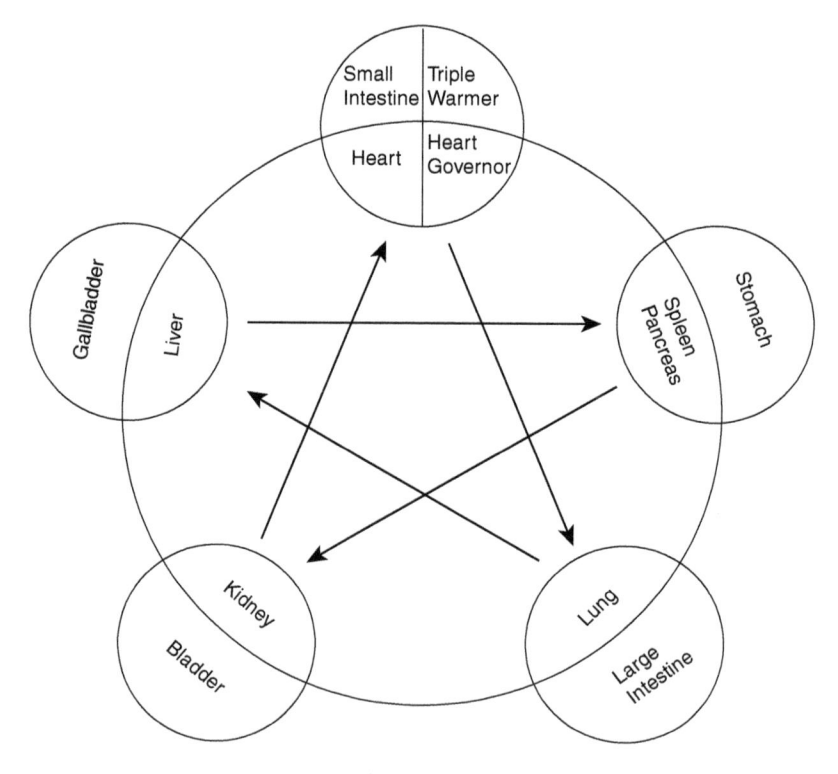

The Ko Cycle

pentagram — the symbol of white magic when it is right-side up, and the symbol of black magic when it is upside down. Like the Shéng cycle, the Ko cycle, the cycle of control, is a system of abstract symbols that makes it possible to connect empirical observations and ideas from very different areas with one another. In the Chinese texts, the laws of the Ko cycle were portrayed in the following manner: water puts out fire, fire melts metal, metal (in the form of a saw or an ax) cuts wood, wood (as a plant or tree) breaks through the surface of the earth, earth dams up the path of water.

Too much water extinguishes the fire completely. One finds this relationship between Water and Fire in people who are ambitious, driven, and strong-willed but who lack warmth, joy, and a bright quality. This can also be seen in people who are full of fear and paranoia; fear is the opponent of love.

Too little water allows the fire to blaze too high. The fire consumes itself too quickly and results in a flash in the pan instead of a warming fire. The consequences on the emotional level are overenthusiasm, mania and hysteria, and carousing and revelry, which turn to depression after the fire has burned out. Other signs of this sort of imbalance are insomnia and unstable moods.

Fire melts metal. Fire is necessary in order to give metal a form, in order to refine it. Practical tools and jewelry can be created. The elasticity and hardness of many metals are dependent upon their temperature; in extreme cold, they become brittle, while in warmer temperatures, they are more flexible and resistant. To the mental qualities of Metal, to the striving for purity and spirituality, the warmth of Fire adds enthusiasm, serenity, cheerfulness, and joy that are characteristic of a truly religious person. Too little Fire leads to zealotry. Too much Fire leads to religious hysteria and rapture, to vagueness and obscurity of the mind; the feeling for what is essential in life is lost. On an emotional level, Fire might be able to cheer up a sad person and get them to smile. A joke often helps one get over low spirits and dejectedness.

Metal cuts wood. The polarity of expansion and contraction, of spring and fall, characterizes this relationship. People with an overly strong Metal give the impression of being withdrawn or cut off and isolated from their surroundings. It often appears as if they are carrying around sadness from their childhood, expressed in their pale complexion. They have a tendency to let their shoulders droop. They are marked by a fearfulness and a pessimistic attitude that block them from making a fresh start and being courageous. It is difficult for them to dedicate themselves to new projects and to meet new people. They don't take the necessary risks to get what they want, and they don't allow themselves to be aggressive. They would rather have their sad face than a thunderstorm that clears the air, and sometimes rationalize this through a religious doctrine.

In contrast, too little Metal allows the Wood to grow wild. This type of person lives expansively and takes on new adventures again and again. Such a person will be full of entrepreneurial spirit and inventiveness but will sometimes become lost in the activities; a sense of what is really important might be lacking at times.

Wood penetrates the earth. If the forest or jungle covers an entire country, then there is hardly any room for fertile fields. If there is no forest, the soil will not be able to hold moisture, the minerals will be washed away, and the country will be transformed into a desert or steppe. Wood is the grandmother of the earth; it is responsible for its fertility. The relationship between Wood and Earth is characterized by the polarity of activity and receptivity. If a person is too active, making too many plans, taking on too many projects, and having too many decisions to make, then many of these projects will not be able to mature, and it will be difficult to find peace within. People who are not rooted may travel a lot or feel as if they are always on the go. This way of life can lead to irritability and insecurity. The Earth element provides a feeling of security. Wood that is too strong brings with it an overall aggressiveness; where there is a lot of aggression, there is little room for empathy and sympathy, little readiness to care for others and to be there for them.

In contrast, if Wood is weak and cannot control the Earth, then a Shí state of the Spleen results: an overprotectiveness of others, an effusive romanticism, or a constant brooding over what one failed to do in life because one did not assert oneself, carry through, and succeed.

Earth cuts off the path of water. The picture of this relationship is a dam that regulates the flow of water. It prevents the water from flooding the land after a heavy rainfall. The interplay between earth and water ensures that there is enough water for the fields for the whole year. On a human level, this expresses itself as the polarity of having both a sense of reality and deep, uncontrollable feelings — the polarity of practicality and reason, mysticism and sensitivity. On the one hand, there is the Earth with its sense of what is important in life, and on the other hand, the element Water with its tendency toward dreams, music, drugs, deep feelings, and sinking into the unconscious.

A person in whom the Earth element is too strong will have priorities, such as keeping the house in order, fulfilling job responsibilities correctly, earning money, and getting recognition. This recognition will be obtained by observing the morals and ethics of the culture, not necessarily because of an inherent feeling of right and wrong or personal values. This focus on material things doesn't leave much room for arriving at a deeper understanding of the Water element, which will be repressed, perhaps through fighting. This type of person often makes sweeping judgments about meditation, hypnosis, drugs, and ecstatic feelings. Fear of one's own suppressed feelings is usually the basis for this kind of behavior.

If the Earth element is too weak and can no longer regulate the flow of Water, it results in a flood of the psyche — a flood of feelings over which one has no control. One gets flooded by strong feelings and becomes afraid of having the rug pulled out from under one's feet. Deep feelings are often accompanied by this fear of losing control over one's life and one's actions. This fear goes away only when one has learned to trust Water and destiny.

If the element Water predominates, it results in a feeling of being at the mercy of society and of not being able to control one's own emotions. Inner turbulence and unreasonable fears can become as strong as a tidal wave. These existential fears are a constituting element in drug addiction, schizophrenia, and psychosis.

The Ko cycle also determines the relationship between Yáng and Yin in the organism. The "grandmother" Yáng organ controls the "grandchild" Yin organ. For example, the Gallbladder controls the Spleen, the Stomach controls the Kidneys, and so on. Hyperfunction and hypofunction of the Gallbladder will adversely affect the energy system of the Spleen Pancreas and, in many cases, damage it. Simply stated, one could say that hyperfunction of the Gallbladder energy leads to a suppression of the energy cycle in the Spleen. With hypofunction, the energy system of the Spleen becomes too strong and thus will also become imbalanced.

The Ko cycle ensures that a balance of energy among the elements can be reached and maintained, in nature and in humans. Through this cycle, the growth of each individual element is limited to such an extent that organic, useful growth can come about.

If one applies the Ko cycle to the emotional level, it becomes clear that the basic human feelings are all equally important — not only for emotional balance but also for the balance and stability of the physical body and the spiritual self — as these three levels are in constant interaction. Annoyance, anger, laughter, joy, sympathy, melancholy, sadness, grief, lust, and fear all are of the same value in our life because they are constitutional energies of ourselves and are the expression of the five elemental forces that create and form our body, mind, and soul. A person whose elements are balanced will be able to feel and follow all of these emotional impulses.

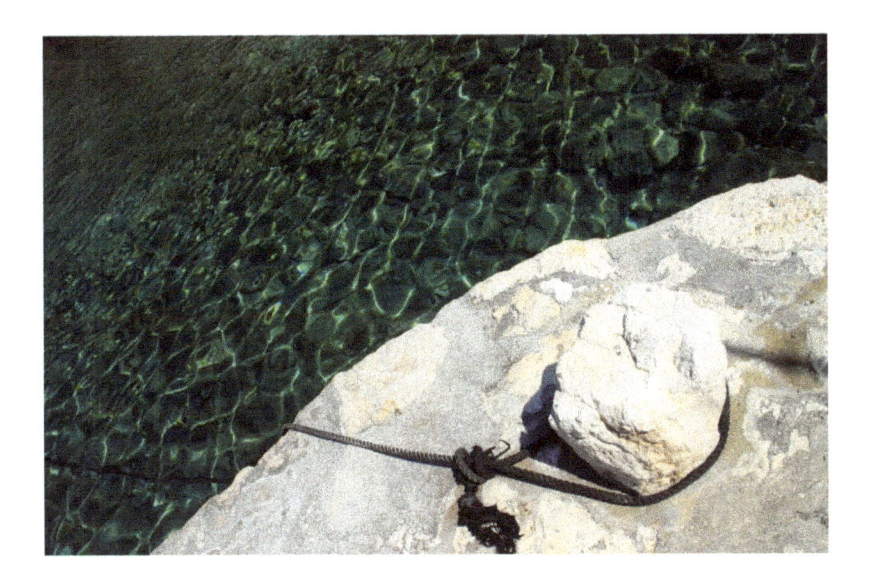

It is obvious that, in our culture, joy and compassion are well received most of the time, while anger, lust, grief, and fear are not. This attitude has far-reaching consequences, as all of the basic emotions that are judged negatively, suppressed, or repressed by an individual or society will, according to the laws of the Shéng and Ko cycles, severely disturb the delicate interplay of the elements. People who never show annoyance and anger may be pleasant to others, but this behavior affects not only their element Wood but also directly affects their Fire and Earth. They will probably show little warmth and spontaneity and will feel very little true joy in life. They try to be pleasant and obliging toward others, but their bodies will express this imbalance. They may tend toward obesity, diabetes, gastritis, or other diseases of the Earth element.

Many analogous examples could be listed. A person who cannot laugh and cry, a person who cannot be furious and fearful, a person who cannot sense the worries of others is missing a power and cannot live life fully. Every one-sided predominance of certain feelings — certain ways of thinking and behavioral patterns — results in an imbalance of the elements. This increases with time and undermines one's well-being, later leading to uneasiness and unhappiness and eventually, when the imbalance is no longer experienced consciously, to chronic physical illnesses. The majority of the diseases of civilization (migraines, back problems, menstrual disorders, high blood pressure, heart attacks, diabetes, and so forth) arise in this way. They develop in a process that takes years or decades. They mirror the uneasiness within this culture, the burden of civilization.

The Cycle of Rebellion

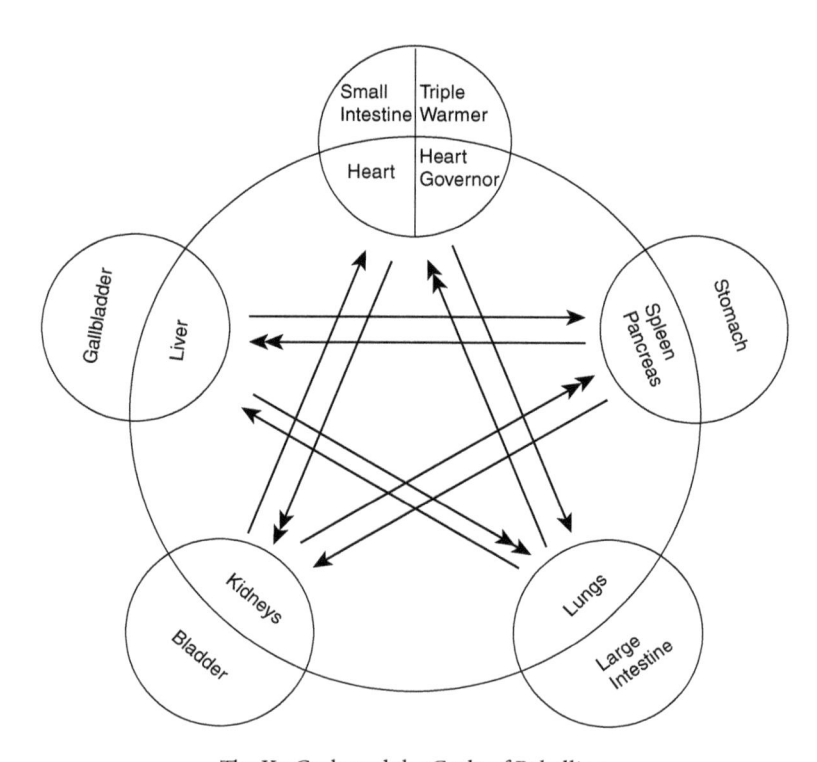

The Ko Cycle and the Cycle of Rebellion

The cycle of rebellion is described in the Chinese tradition as the "grandchild who rebels against the grandmother."

If too much energy is in Wood, then Wood first damages Earth (through the Ko cycle). However, an overly strong Wood could also rebel against Metal and bring this element out of balance. That is the relationship of the strong, impudent grandchild to its grandmother; the grandchild has lost respect for the grandmother and therefore confronts her methods of upbringing.

A surplus of Wood can create an illness in the Earth element as well as an illness or disturbance in Metal. This is how a person whose attention is basically directed toward work and career, who constantly has to prevail, maintain a position of power, and make precise decisions will display an imbalance in Metal. In later years, such a person may be incapable of giving up the identity of the successful entrepreneur, breaking down and dying soon after retirement, or being incapable of grief or tears.

The Cycle of Withdrawal

This law is rather graphically described as the "child who damages the mother" or as the "greedy child who sucks the mother dry."

If the energy of an element has been constantly used up by a bad habit, by unbalanced character traits, or by particular stress on this element because of chronic illness, then too much energy can be withdrawn from the nourishing mother element via the Shéng cycle. Then, the mother herself becomes weak and sick. To give an example, through a sedentary life, constant reading, brooding, thinking, or a chronic Earth element illness, not only is the Earth weakened but also Fire, because the Earth, using up more energy than is available within the Earth element, takes the missing energy from the mother — as long as it is there. The child sucks the mother dry. This can, under certain circumstances, also lead to an illness of the Fire element. The mother who spends half her life taking care of her family, who constantly has to sympathize with everyone, will eventually lose her *joie de vivre* if she does not have a strong personality and inner resources. Another

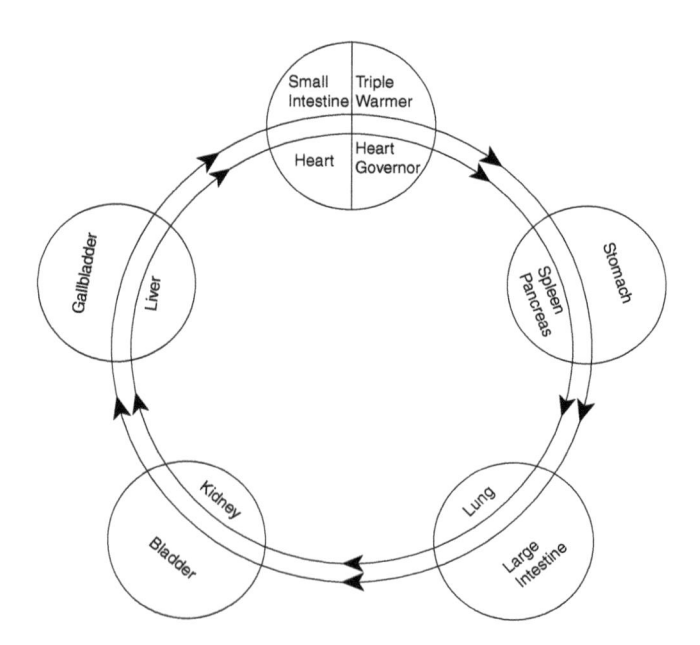

The Cycle of Withdrawal

example would be the civil servant or bookkeeper who loses more zest for life with every year spent doing the same thing.

The following example clarifies the role that the four cycles can play in the emergence of an illness. In many cases, a lung disease will be directly due to an emotional or physiological imbalance in Metal. However, the same lung disease can also arise from an imbalance in the Spleen ("the mother does not give the child enough nourishment"). It can come about through sick Kidneys ("the child withdraws energy from the mother"). Also, an imbalance in the Fire element — a heart defect or arteriosclerosis — can cause lung disease ("the grandmother is too soft or too hard on the grandchild"). Eventually, it can arise from an imbalance in Wood ("the grandchild rebels against the grandmother").

With this example, one can see how important an exact diagnosis of the cause of a disease is, as this diagnosis determines the starting point of therapy. Hence, chronic bronchitis will sometimes be treated through Earth, in another case through Fire, and in yet another case through the Lungs and Large Intestine, the Metal organs.

The element from which the illness or imbalance arises can be detected through the fine methods of diagnostics that are a part of Chinese medicine. Diagnosis is beyond the scope of this book, but suffice it to say that chronic symptoms can only be healed when one has found the original cause of the disorder and treated it.

Serious and acute symptoms, such as high fever, circulatory collapse, or intense pain, almost always require a direct, "symptomatic" treatment first, especially when the situation is life-threatening. Only afterward can a doctor attend to the cause of the disorder.

The success of traditional Chinese medicine in treating chronic illnesses is, for the most part, based on restoring the balance of the elements. In many cases, this is possible via knowledge of the four cycles and help from suitable therapeutic methods: diet, herbal extracts, breathing and physical exercises, meridian massage, Shiatsu, acupressure, acupuncture, and meditation.

Practical Use of the Cycles

This section on the four cycles can help you to make the right decision when choosing the exercises that best correspond to your needs. You will also be able to understand and interpret events and experiences in your life when you perform the exercises regularly.

The sequence of the exercises is also important. It is advantageous to arrange the exercises according to the Shéng cycle, beginning with Wood and ending with Water. This is relevant if you do all or most of the exercises — the emotional and mental as well as the physical exercises. If you decide to explore the nature of the Five Elements, start by doing the exercises for the element that seems to be weakest in your personality. If it is not obvious with which element to start, start with Wood. Focus on each element, in the order of the

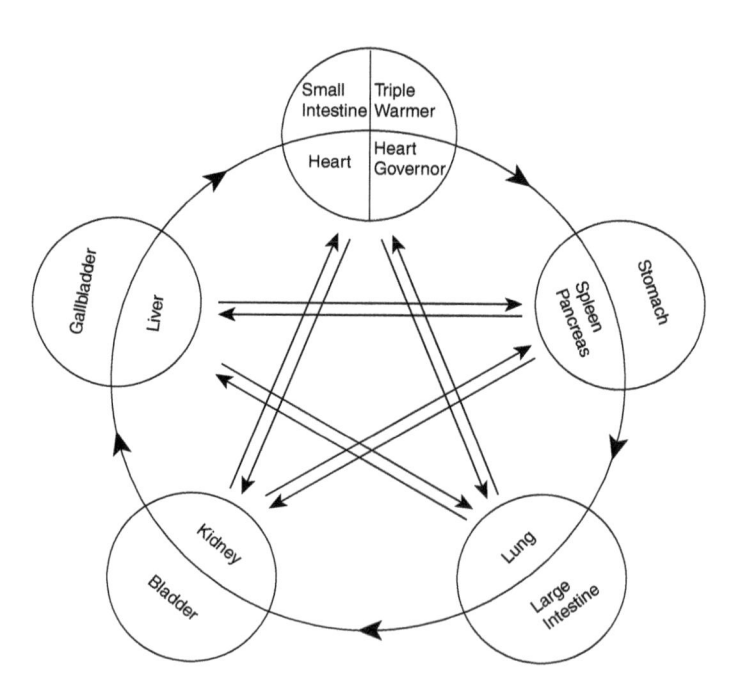

The Shéng and Ko Cycles, and the Cycle of Rebellion

Shéng cycle, for some time — maybe for a week or two — to really experience the individual quality and power of each element.

In merely doing the physical exercises that stimulate energy flow through the organs and their meridians, it is recommended that you proceed in the order of the Qì flow through the meridians. The circulation of Qì in the Twelve Organ Meridians has its own sequence. It is different from the laws of the four cycles described in this chapter. Qì flows in the meridians in the following order: from Lung to Large Intestine to Stomach to Spleen to Heart to Small Intestine to Bladder to Kidney to Pericardium to Triple Warmer to Gallbladder to Liver — and from the Liver Meridian, the circulating Qì flows back to the Lung Meridian to start a new cycle. The circulation of Qì in the body is a continuous flow similar to the blood circulation.

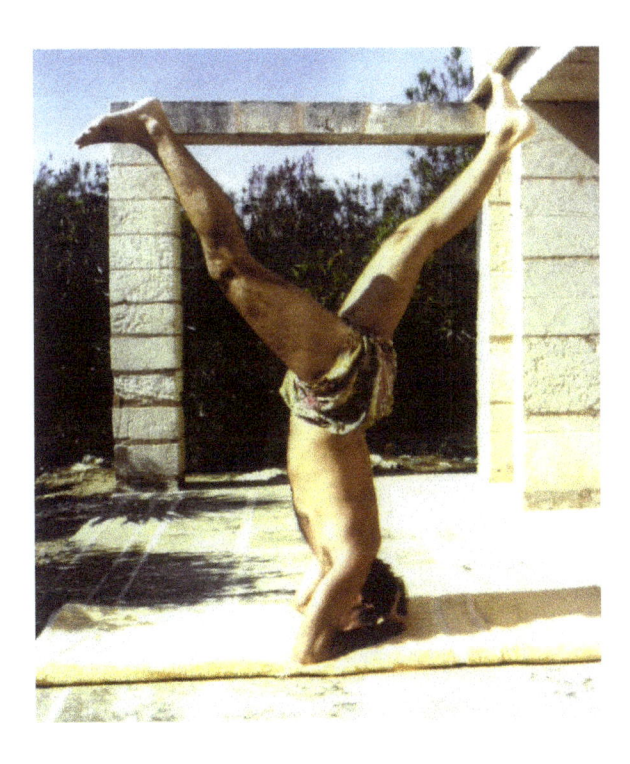

If you want to enhance your energy to get going for the day, to feel healthy and alive, do physical exercises to stimulate the Qì How in the meridians. As in working with the elements, select the meridian exercises of those organs that seem to be weaker than others. Select between six and twelve exercises, and pause after each posture for a moment with your eyes closed to feel the specific effect.

Epilogue

Every time period and every culture has its Achilles' heel. The Achilles' heel of the twentieth century is the continual poisoning of our planet and its atmosphere and the ever-growing threat posed to nature by humans who, through our search for prosperity and material security, are destroying the basic support systems needed for our lives and those of the plants and other animals. Technology and civilized living, created to protect us from natural catastrophes, have gotten the upper hand to the extent that things are out of balance. We are now left with the question of how we can protect ourselves from technology and civilization.

In the eighteenth and nineteenth centuries, class differences and contrasts in the standard of living were a source of tension in social structures in Europe and the United States. These disparities led to enormous changes and revolutions, from the French Revolution to the growth of communism in Eastern Europe. In the second half of the twentieth century, ecological problems have pushed their way to the forefront. In these times, in Europe and North America, the confrontation between humans and nature has become as important as the confrontations among human beings, if not more so.

The Earth is a living being — an enormous organism, say the Native American Hopi Tribe. In the twentieth century, it is sick, and the nature spirits have withdrawn into the Earth. It is possible that the Earth will cramp up and shake itself loose until she can once again breathe freely.

Humanity can be seen as the Brain of the Earth, the carrier of a certain form of intelligence and rationality; humans are the gray and white ganglion cells of the Earth organism. The ganglion cells are capable of learning very quickly from each other and passing on their experiences to other parts of the nervous system. They are capable of imagining changes and manifesting them, thereby influencing and changing other parts of the organism.

It is similar in the human organism. Humans are capable of following their intellect, even when it is not in the best interest of the body. A child can be so fascinated by the discovery of the world of its mind that it forgets everything else around it. The more it reads and thinks, the more it will feel at home in the world of ideas. Eventually, it will consider its thoughts to be reality; the ideas it has about life become life itself. At some point, it will take it one step further and no longer trust its own senses if these speak against the concept it has built up in its mind.

One can compare how most people in Western cultures treat their bodies with how most of humanity treats the Earth. Many people in the West no longer know how it feels to be *in* their bodies, to be a body. They do not know what it is like to perceive the world directly with their senses. They *have* a body, but they are not this body. They confuse thinking about life with life itself.

Just as Western medicine is helpless in the face of many chronic diseases of civilization, we also feel helpless in regard to making decisions about our dying forests and other environmental disasters. Our society is just as powerless in trying to stop cancer, AIDS, arteriosclerosis, diabetes, arthritis, allergies, and skin diseases as it is in trying to stop the destruction of rivers, forests, and the soil through chemical products, heavy metals, and radioactivity. We have not yet come to our senses, or we would have revolted a long time ago.

What should we do? Where should we begin? How can we turn back the clock to a time when people were not separate from nature, to a time when there was no split between body and soul? There are only a few people in the world today who are aware of the dimensions of these problems. At best, one can expect a form of plastic surgery from the leaders in government, industry, and education, and unfortunately no real change in thought or behavior. Only an ecological catastrophe would force them to quickly and thoroughly change their way of thinking and replace the mostly material goals of our prosperity-minded society with goals that are more in tune with life on this planet.

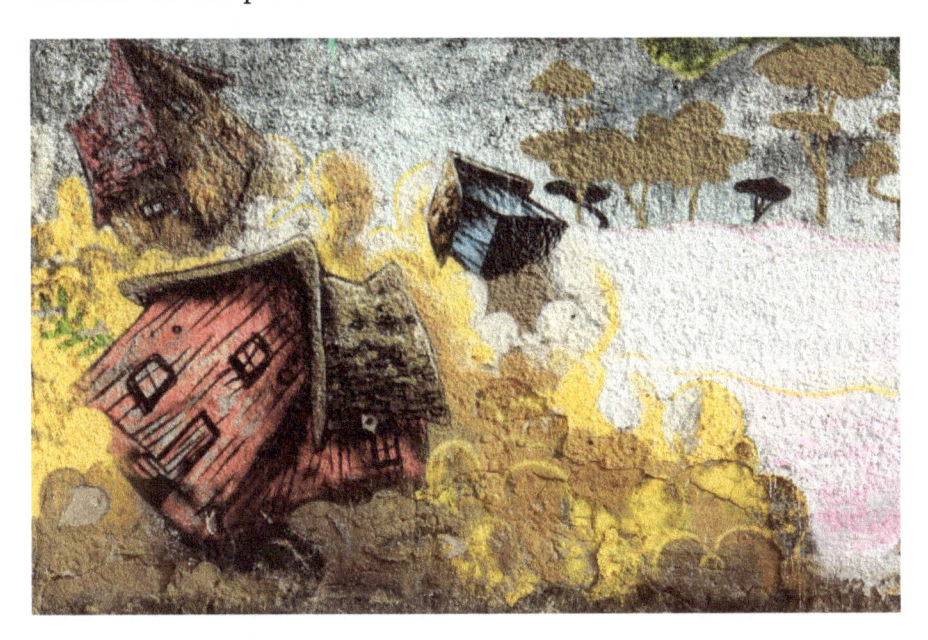

What to do? How can we save the planet? What position do we have to take to help to save the planet? What things do we have to refrain from doing? Can we wait for our politicians and environmental conferences to come to decisions? It seems that the political system that would have to pass effective laws to reduce the emissions of carbon dioxide, to reduce the poisoning of the rivers and of the sea, to save the ozone layer, and so forth is worldwide, except maybe in countries like Bhutan and Nepal, to such an extent in the grip of the various economic lobbies that the measures taken so far against the global pollution and the disintegration of the Earth's biological systems are totally inadequate and incomplete. As the situation is today, can we wait for our politicians to do this enormous job to pass hundreds of environmental laws that totally go against the ways and the ideals of the affluent society? It seems that our politicians are not able to do it. One of the reasons might be that they only are the tip of the iceberg — the iceberg being the Judao-Christian culture stream which turned against nature already 3,000 years ago, which decided that man should be separate from the plant and animal kingdoms and the Earth be made a subject. Read the Bible, it's all in there, it's all said in the story of the Creation. Now we have to deal with the consequences.

It seems that our politicians — and that really means our whole Western culture — do not have the foresight (an ability of the Liver) together with the power (an ability of, mainly, the Gallbladder, Stomach, and Spleen but also of the Kidney as our will to survive) to change the course of environmental destruction fast.

What to do? It seems that we have to rely on ourselves.

But what to do? Most of us do not have the power to bring a dead river back to life. Most of us do not have the power to force industries to be more conscious of nature. Most of us are not able to get rid of our poisonous cars, lorries, and planes overnight. Our economy has become so complex and the individual branches so dependant on each other that each sudden change threatens our survival instincts. But these survival instincts have been shaped in a different environment, in a different age. What helped us then can destroy us tomorrow. But our basic security patterns are not that clever. It seems that we have to gather all intelligence to come to new — or very old — solutions fast.

What can we do? How can we undo our separation from nature? On the one hand, we can put all of our energy into seeing that changes occur. We can change ourselves and our lives so that we use fewer consumer goods and do without vicarious satisfaction. We can buy fewer cars and only one TV set and one video recorder per family, we can drive less often, eat less meat, and take fewer pharmaceutical products. We can choose new goals that satisfy our body, mind, and soul in equal measure — goals that are not as destructive to the environment. We can learn to give each other a massage instead of driving to the disco forty miles away on Saturday night. Or we can, every now and then, adopt the attitude of riding a bicycle to do some errands instead of doing our workout on the home trainer or in the fitness center and using the car to drive three blocks. And we have heard many of these suggestions.

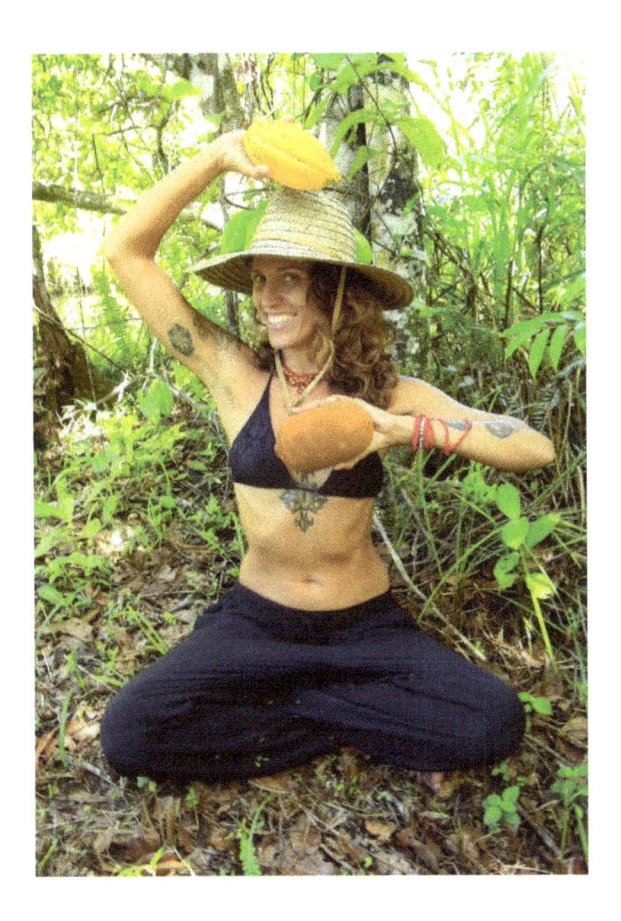

On the other hand, it seems that we have to change a bit more than a few of our deeds and actions. It seems that we also have to undergo an inner process to become reconciled with nature in ourselves. It seems that we have to make our peace with nature. Earth is the Mother, not an enemy. It seems that we have to become reconciled with our emotions, with our fantasies and dreams, with our spiritual being. If we are not in tune with nature in ourselves, how can we act in the outside world to save the planet? As long as we fight the animal part in ourselves, how can we sincerely develop the sympathy necessary to save all the endangered species? As long as we forget about the plant part in ourselves — that quiescent and meditative part — how can we develop the love necessary to fight for all the endangered species?

It seems that, as we are all parts of the "iceberg," we need to start trusting nature again, we need to become again familiar with the elements. And it seems that we also have to start with ourselves, spending more time fulfilling the basic needs of our body and soul in order to make a return to the essence of life possible.

The Dào of Healing in Times of War and Pandemic

Five-Element thinking

In most ancient cultures, theoretical systems to explain the world originated in the observation of nature, and in most cases, these systems evolved into religious beliefs and into scientific thinking.

In many cultures, basic principles or gods are derived from forces of nature: wind and thunder, heat and sun, moisture and fertility, dryness and sky, coldness and rain. The ancient Chinese observed that climate factors can be attributed to seasons: winds in spring, heat in the summer, moisture in late summer, dryness in fall, and coldness in winter.

The law of the Five Elements can be applied to understanding cycles of growth and decay in nature as well as in economic, sociological, and political structures. The contemporary dictate of economic growth at all costs and the fear of recession clearly show that modern societies are out of kilter with the basic laws of nature.

Human beings have existed for a million years. For most of that time, we were hunter-gatherers who lived in symbiosis with nature. Human beings do not have the claws and teeth of a tiger or a lion nor the muscular strength and running speed of other beasts of prey, so they invented the technique of burning down the woods to be able to hunt the fleeing animals successfully. Thus, by burning down forests on a large scale to ensure their own survival, hunter-gatherers changed the face of the earth.

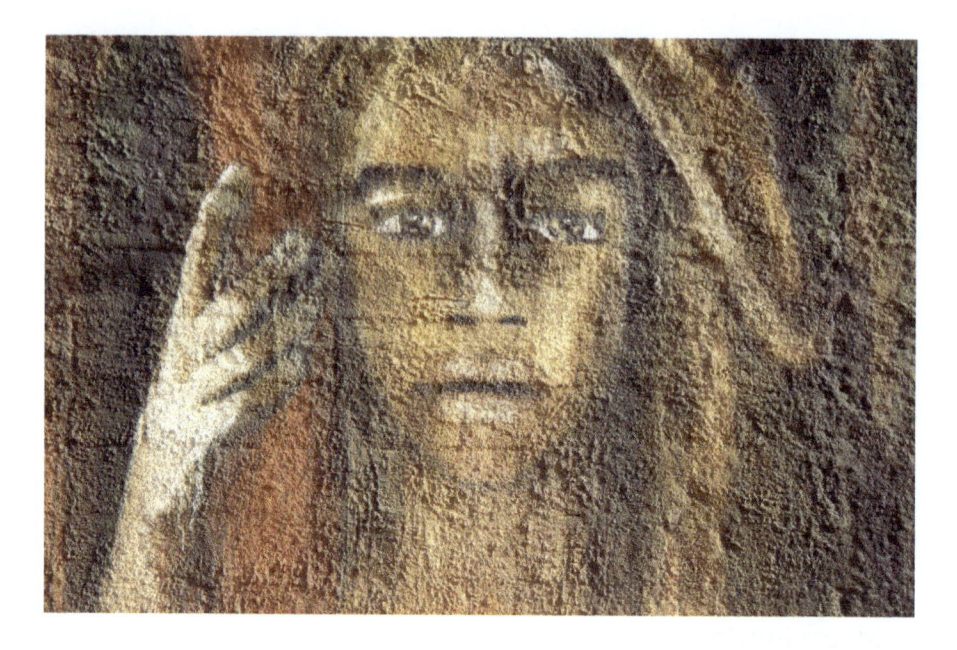

Agricultural societies have existed for about 10,000 years. Likewise, woods were cut down to gain arable land to sow and harvest — to survive on agricultural crops.

The process of burning down the forests and transforming greenfield sites for economic exploitation has not slowed down in recent years, and green spaces are being reduced at an enormous speed. Untouched nature seems to exist only in national parks. (Thus once again, nature is being exploited as an economic commodity.) The anaerobic metabolism of mammals developed in symbiosis with endless forests that absorb carbon dioxide and produce oxygen. If forests disappear, mammals will also disappear. Right now, every 15 minutes an animal species goes extinct. Every 15 minutes the evolutionary achievement of hundred million years is being sacrificed for our greed, to possess as much as possible, as fast as possible. Every 15 minutes another wonder of evolution is destroyed.

The rainforests of the Amazon and of Indonesia also serve the function of cooling down the planet. They are Mother Earth's giant air conditioning system. We are already noticing a significant heating up of the climate, long periods of dryness in many parts of the world, recently especially in Australia, California, and many African and European countries. On the other hand, excessive rainfalls lead to floods and deluges that damage cities and destroy agricultural land.

I wonder why the very rich people of the world and the governments of wealthy states do not just buy the rain forests of the Amazon, the Congo and Borneo, and Java and Sumatra? What is the use of spending billions on developing vaccines or cancer treatments, or to produce arms and travel into space, billions to grout the world, when we already know that this road will lead to a miserable end in the near future?

We know that we consume too much. We know that we need to eat less meat and more local products. We know that we are buying too many clothes and habitually buying new things instead of repairing them.

The COVID-19 pandemic and the increasing prices for oil and gas during the Russian-Ukrainian war brought some restrictions on mobility, traveling, and general consumer habits. Instead of taking the opportunity to correct and downsize our consuming habits, the governments in European states spent again billions to enable people to continue driving and spending.

For the last 1,000 years, Western culture has emphasized the force of Wood. Conquering and subduing other cultures, developing woods and meadows, mountains and rivers, lakes and seas into structures that only serve our needs but violate nature in millions of ways.

The principle of permanent economic growth has to be maintained at all costs. Modern societies only function if there is permanent growth. In the laws of the Five Elements, this means excess of Wood that rebels against Metal, Eternal Spring against Fall.

Fall depicts the essence of Metal: concentration and condensation; the energy is directed within. Principles of metal are moderation, restriction, confining, recession, moving less, and spending less.

In the Ko cycle, excessive Wood breaks the Earth. We can see that on all continents Mother Earth is being broken constantly at the speed of light, with the growing of electric cables all over.

Now, the fear of blackout. Blackout is inevitable and also necessary. No civilization can grow indefinitely. Metal cuts Wood. The extent of economic growth during the last 200 years since the beginning of the industrial age will be matched by the recession following it to bring the interplay of elementary forces on the planet into balance again. Modern science and urbanization have made possible two radical schemes that might end the height of human civilization. One is a nuclear war which would freeze the planet and kill parts of humanity as well as a lot of infrastructure, production sites, and transport systems thus reducing the further thriving of consumer capitalism. The other one is future endemics that result in the destruction of natural habitats so that many animals with their inherent viruses need to live in cities. As a result, the human immune system is weakened by too many toxic substances and too much microplastic in the body, and too little contact with nature to develop a natural immune force (spending two hours in a forest strengthens the immune system measurably for a week) — a breeding ground for future endemics. There are also too many vaccines — which do a lot of good if used against specific strong killers like tetanus and smallpox, but which confuse and weaken the immune system when they are given against antigens that could be mastered by the proper immune system. The over-vaccination of humanity in the last 50 years has been a success for the pharmaceutical industry, but it has led to the reality that today over a third of the human population is suffering from over-reacting immune responses commonly called allergies. In the early 1960s, about 3% of humanity suffered from allergies.

From history, we know that there are good and bad governments, to put it simply. There are governments that care for the well-being of their citizens, while others focus on the well-being of a small upper class only.

We can easily imagine that in future resources like water, oxygen, nutrition, certain elements like antimony, silver, lithium, and rare earths but also simple things like sand for construction sites will become more and more scarce for a still growing humanity. One of the major driving forces for modern humanity is greed, and we can imagine that at some point an oligarchy is capable of reducing the number of consumers of dwindling resources by rather surreptitious methods. One very elegant method is making vaccination which can kill (or "not help") parts of the population mandatory. Vaccines can contain a number of different substances. How can we know what they contain?

Even if a minority of scientists find out what is going on, we have seen during the COVID-19 pandemic, especially in Europe, that all voices that promote alternative methods to combat the pandemic or warn of the side effects of mRNA vaccines were discredited, ridiculed, and showered with public anger. In some countries, such as Italy, Germany, and Austria, doctors, healers, and pharmacists who treated COVID-19 with methods other than vaccination sometimes even lost their license. In Austria, one in nine million of the population refused to have the COVID-19 vaccination.

Some people rely on other medical systems like Traditional Chinese Medicine (TCM), orthomolecular therapy, homeopathy, and Ayurveda, or on cheap, but effective drugs, like Ivermectin.

Ivermectin is a drug which kills invertebrates. Thus, it is used with people as well as domestic animals and cattle to eliminate parasites. The WHO propagated the drug to treat river blindness (caused by filaria) in about 100 million people, especially in Africa and also South America. Ivermectin has been used in humans since the 1980s. Over four billion doses have been administered. Merck, the original patent holder, donated 3.7 billion doses to developing countries. In 2015, William C. Campbell and Satoshi Ōmura, who developed Ivermectin, were awarded the Nobel Prize for Medicine. While known primarily as an anti-parasitic, Ivermectin also has anti-viral and anti-inflammatory properties. Evidence shows that Ivermectin was given to about 350 million of the residents in the Indian states of Uttar Pradesh, Uttarakhand, Goa, and Karnataka in May 2021 to break the tide of the COVID-19-pandemic, and figures show that in those states the peak of the pandemic was broken much faster than in other Indian states which did not hand out the drug for everybody as a preventive measure.[1]

The patent of Merck on Ivermectin expired in 1996. There is no more money to be made from this drug. Any country can produce it cheaply. That's why there are a lot of warnings about and advice against Ivermectin on the internet — a good example of how science today follows money. European countries with their high standards of care for their citizens are the golden cash cow of Big Pharma, and as a result, the work of the Big Pharma lobby is very fierce in Europe. Those whose opinion relies only on what they find on the internet at first sight can be manipulated easily.

The author got infected with SARS-CoV-2 in South America. The symptoms were fever, feeling sick with no energy, and a few days

---

[1] https://www.indiatoday.in/coronavirus-outbreak/story/ivermectin-tablet-uttarakhand-residents-prevent-covid-govt-1801863-2021-05-12; https://www.biznews.com/thought-leaders/2021/05/12/mailbox-ivermectin.

later a strong cough. With the combination of Chinese herbal teas, Ivermectin, acupressure points of the Lungs, Heart, and Spleen-Pancreas, and further the Ayurvedic practice of inhaling hot steam twice a day for about a minute, he was able to shake off the infection within a few days. On Day 4, he was able to do a 45-minute walk in 30°C heat in the afternoon. On Day 6, he was able to run a mile in 30°. The cost of the treatment was about 50 euros: 30 euros for Ivermectin and 20 euros for Nanking Tea Nr 1 and Nr 2.

That's not going to fill the coffers of Big Pharma.

Others in Austria knew friends or family members who suffered from sometimes severe side effects after the vaccination. Side effects are widespread and can affect any organ, including the Heart, the Arteries, the Brain, the Lungs, and the Intestines. The reason is that the messenger RNA of an mRNA vaccine simulates the existence of an original DNA segment that orders the ribosomes (the protein factories of the cell) to produce the spike protein of SARS-CoV-2. The existence of the spike protein in the body alarms the immune system and fosters the various immune responses. So far nobody knows how long the mRNA of the vaccine remains in the body. As long as it remains and wherever it accumulates, it triggers an alarm reaction in the body and may cause an immune response against the cells of any organ.

The widespread side effects have shown that autoimmune responses may occur in any organ and tissues and that they predominantly occur in pre-damaged organs or arteriosclerotic blood vessels leading to thrombosis and embolism. Side effects can be severe and include myocarditis and sudden heart failure, or just lead to ongoing weakness and being unable to run 50 yards without a pumping heartbeat and the feeling of exhaustion. In a few years, we will see whether the prevalence of cancer has also increased significantly because the immune system of many people was disturbed by too many vaccinations in a short period of time. In cell division, cancer cells constantly emerge. Our immune system is only able to eliminate the cancer cells if it is in good balance.

BKK Benchmark, the biggest health insurance provider in Germany with about 11 million insured persons (13% of the German population), stated that in 2021 they paid the treatments of 216,695 patients because of side effects of the COVID-19 vaccination. These are over 2% of the insured. As many people got treatments for disorders and diseases which were not recognized by doctors to be related to the previous COVID-19 vaccination, and as many people with minor disorders like sleeplessness, headaches, anxiety, shortness of breath, and fatigue after the vaccination did not go to get medical help, but treated these symptoms on their own with sleeping pills, pain killers, tranquilizers, etc., we can estimate that at least 5% of the vaccinated are suffering from some form of side effects — one in 20. BKK Benchmark stated that in 2021 they paid for the treatment of 7,748 people suffering from side effects of all other vaccinations. This means that the COVID-19 vaccination caused 30 times more side effects than all other vaccinations in Germany in 2021.

The CEO of BKK Benchmark did his duty to publish these figures and was promptly forced to resign by the German health minister — another example of how often science today is not primarily about truth but about the need to follow economic requirements and demands. Research of scientists can only be acknowledged and published if the findings do not disturb the flow of cash to the rich.

As a result of many people living healthier lives, sales of medicine declined in the last decades. Then comes the COVID-19 pandemic and Big Pharma used it well and effectively to discredit Traditional Chinese Medicine, homeopathy, Ayurveda, and common herbal treatments against infections of the upper respiratory tract.

Countries like India were much more successful in combating the pandemic than European countries or the US, as they combined the vaccination with all other medical systems and medicaments available: Ivermectin, Ayurveda, homeopathy, and Traditional Chinese Medicine. Traditional Chinese Medicine was very successful in China in the early months of the pandemic, before vaccination became available.

Chinese and Western allopathic medicine during the pandemic

Two things were not addressed in the course of the public debate during the COVID-19 pandemic in Europe: how to prevent an infection of the upper respiratory tract using "home remedies" and how the general health of those most at risk could be improved in order to prevent a more severe progression of COVID-19.

We know that obesity, diabetes, arteriosclerosis, and related cardiovascular diseases are underlying health conditions that can lead to a more severe progression of COVID-19. However, in European countries, there were no public campaigns to enhance the positive impact fitness or better nutrition can have on the respiratory system, circulation, or the immune system.

It's almost as if whooping cough, tuberculosis, angina, influenza, chronic bronchitis, or asthma had never existed. Since the beginning of time, human beings have taken herbs in the form of tea or as an extract, inhaled their active healing substances in a steam bath, or rubbed them into their skin in the form of oils so that they could reach their Lungs and mucous membranes via the bloodstream.

Those in the UK, Austria, or Germany who had tested positive for COVID-19 had to wait until the infection had passed or until it got so bad that they had to be taken to hospital. Self-isolation was the only measure recommended.

In the four weeks leading up to 26 February 2022, more than 57% of new infections with SARS-CoV-2 worldwide happened in Europe. Europe, including Ukraine, Russia, and Turkey, has a population of 750 million — in contrast to the rest of the world with more than seven billion people. In November 2021, well above half of all new infections globally occurred in Europe. How did Europe, despite its pandemically incessant propaganda through the media, its often strict measures of self-isolation or lockdown, and its comparatively high average vaccination rate, manage to become the global leader when it came to the rate of infection?

In my view, the medical and pharmaceutical lobby has managed with the help of "studies" by the WHO to ban all preclinical forms of therapy from the fight against the pandemic in Europe, to ignore them, ridicule them, or to forbid them. The most important among them are probably TCM, orthomolecular therapy, homeopathy, and Ayurveda.

In the four weeks leading up to 6 January 2022, Great Britain with its population of 67.6 million and 70.8% double-vaccinated came second in the world league table with 3.246.972 new infections. A long way behind was India in 13th place: A population of 1400 million, of whom 56.7% had had their first vaccination and 30.6% had by then received a second dose. India had 443,045 new infections. Thus in the four weeks leading up to 6 January 2022, India had 13.6% of the new infections of Great Britain, while having a far lower vaccination rate and twenty times the population.

It's not merely a matter of the vaccination rate but also of the use of preclinical medications and therapies, which are particularly widespread in India. There are ayurvedic and homeopathic clinics, and many hospitals have a TCM department.

Integrative medicine

At the beginning of the pandemic in February 2020 in Wuhan, there were half a million people infected with SARS-CoV-2. As of 2020, there were no vaccines for the treatment of COVID-19, patients were increasingly treated with TCM. Like the Hubei Provincial Hospital for Chinese and Western Medicine in Wuhan, across China there are many hospitals where Western medicine is used alongside TCM in the treatment of the same patients.

In 2020, as long as there were no vaccines, more than 50% of all patients in China who tested positive for SARS-CoV-2 had been treated with a combination of TCM and Western medicine. From the very beginning, traditional herbal mixtures, cupping, moxibustion, and acupuncture were an integral part of the national clinical guidelines for the treatment of COVID-19 patients alongside the possibilities of therapy offered by conventional medicine. TCM is able to prevent in many cases severe progressions of COVID-19 so that they don't occur in the first place; it can also alleviate already existing severe symptoms and thus significantly lower the death rate.

When the vaccines were available in 2021, the use of TCM was neglected. India showed that the best result in fighting the pandemic was the combination of vaccination, Ayurveda, homeopathy, TCM, and other methods of natural medicine. China, it seems, wanted to show the superiority of its pharmaceutical industry using vaccination alone for most people, with the result that the pandemic flamed up again several times, when it already was finished in most parts of the world.

TCM diagnostics

TCM diagnostics organizes symptoms on the basis of "climate factors," such as heat, cold, wind, moisture, dryness, and combinations of these "climate factors," such as wind-cold, wind-heat, or moisture-cold. Pulse diagnostics can identify the energetic shape of the Twelve Organs at twelve different pulse points on both wrists. Following an identification of the symptoms as well as pulse and tongue diagnostics, a diagnosis can be made and subsequently relevant herbal mixtures change be chosen and prescribed; cupping, moxibustion, or acupuncture can be used on the acupuncture points relevant to the symptoms. In moxibustion, individual points or meridians are heated up with a glowing cigarette of mugwort (*Artemisia vulgaris*).

Qing Fei Pai Du Tang (QFPDD)

Qing Fei Pai Du Tang (QFPDD) is one of the herbal mixtures that has proved useful in the alleviation of COVID-19 symptoms. In 2020, the Fuwai Hospital in Wuhan conducted a study giving QFPDD to 8,939 patients of whom 2,565 (28.7%) were given QFPDD. In this group, the mortality was 1.2%; in the other group which didn't receive QFPDD, 4.8% died.

The study also found out that through the giving of QFPDD, the mortality rate could be lowered by three-quarters but also that by giving this herbal mixture one could avoid the damage to Liver and Kidneys that often occurs as a side effect of strong medicaments. The results of this study were published in the journal *Phytomedicine*, published by the Dutch publisher Elsevier, on 31 March 2021.

Chinese phytotherapy

QFPDD is only one among many herbal mixtures that have been used successfully in the treatment of COVID-19. A team from Shanghai University of Traditional Chinese Medicine also published the results of their research in May 2021 in volume 85 of the journal *Phytomedicine.*

The article summarizes the studies of more than 300 pharmacologists, biochemists, physiologists, and doctors listed in the appendix of the study. The main aim of the study was to evaluate through which biochemical and physiological mechanisms the herbs used in the treatment of COVID-19 limit inflammation and tissue damage of individual organs and reduce oxidative stress and apoptosis. Apoptosis is a physiological process by which the cell destroys itself, a suicide program pre-programmed in human DNA, which takes place if the cell gets too old, but also if the DNA is damaged — and also in the course of an inflammation that can be initiated by natural killer cells and other macrophages.

The Chinese scientists completed a mammoth task. The many studies were sponsored by the Essential Drug Research and Development and National Key R&D Program of the Ministry for Science and Technology in China, the Hundred Talents Program of the Shanghai Municipal Health Commission, as well as the Three Years Action Plan to Accelerate the Development of Traditional Chinese Medicine. The studies presented the state of research about the pharmacological mechanism of action of the individual herbs. But with considerable arrogance, we claim that TCM isn't a form of evidence-based medicine. Interestingly enough, in spring 2020, some articles with this degrading assertion were published "on the basis of a study conducted by the WHO" in some European countries. The groups on which the studies were conducted were allegedly too small. A QFPDD study with 8,939 patients was considered too small?

Alongside rigorous self-isolation measures, the combination of Western medicine with TCM made a decisive contribution to the containment of the pandemic in China. Between August and October 2020, no further infections were registered in China. Everyday life returned to normal; there were huge parties and an Oktoberfest in Qingdao with hundreds of thousands of visitors without a virus outbreak. When, however, some patients in a hospital in Qingdao tested positive for COVID-19 which had been brought in by a group of travelers, the entire population of 10 million was tested within a few days.

Whenever there are new infections in a province, entire cities are ordered to isolate. At the same time, many are treated with TCM, even as a preventative measure.

TCM in the treatment of COVID-19 and Long COVID

An estimated 1.3 million Brits, i.e. 2% of the population, suffered for more than four weeks from the effects of a SARS-CoV-2 infection, frequently defined as Long COVID. Which preclinical therapies could be used to reduce the number of cases of Long COVID? Peilin Sun, a Chinese doctor and head of a research group, writes in his book *The Pathogenesis and Treatment of COVID-19 and Long COVID with Traditional Chinese Medicine* that he had originally wanted to publish something about the treatment of Long COVID, but then recognized that Long COVID only occurs when COVID-19 in its acute phase wasn't treated properly with TCM. In a book of 704 pages, he presents his research team's results, how COVID-19 is treated with herbs, cupping, moxibustion, and acupuncture. He writes that he regards TCM as one of the best options for the treatment of COVID-19, "but that one should acknowledge that vaccinations are also good measures for preventing infections and the reduction of severe courses of the disease and cases of deaths."

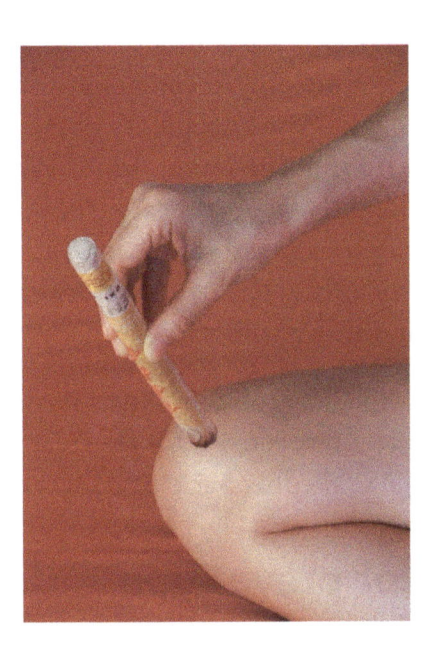

TCM in Europe

In Europe, TCM is a largely untapped resource in the fight against the pandemic. China took our medicine in its entirety and assimilated it. Each medicinal plant has next to its Chinese name the official botanical name in Latin. In a pragmatic way, they apply the type of medicine that is best for the respective situation or disease, or they combine TCM with Western medicine.

TCM is represented in many European countries, predominantly in Great Britain, Germany, Austria, and Switzerland, and also in France, the Netherlands, Belgium, and Sweden. Is it a matter of our cultural arrogance that we tolerate a system of medicine familiar to us and available merely as an exotic plant on the margins, but not to integrate it into our practical work in the hospitals? Or are we simply cash cows of Big Pharma and therefore skilfully misinformed about all other systems of healing?

The price of a herbal mixture is between 6 and 50 euros per week, and an acupuncture needle costs about 5 cents. Therefore, TCM is an affordable medicine, not only in China but also in poor countries, like India and Sri Lanka. For Europe, it's obviously too cheap, Big Pharma is well aware that the countries of Western and Central Europe with their highly developed systems of social care and health insurance are prepared to spend money on the well-being of their citizens and that they have extensive experience in spending money that doesn't exist and never will.

By comparison, drugs like Molnupravir or Paxlovid, developed by Merck & Co. and Pfizer respectively for the treatment of COVID-19 cost approximately 1,000 euros per treatment cycle.

Using TCM for prevention

It is well known that those suffering from obesity, heart, or lung disease are much more severely affected by COVID-19 than those who are healthy. In a healthy society, this could be regarded as an incentive to encourage the entire population to exercise more, to eat less, and to rest more. An open and mentally healthy society would raise greater awareness of different methods of healing that are able to improve health and strengthen the immune system and to make them affordable to the wider population.

Should it not be the task of the ministries of health to investigate all available methods of healing and to prove their effectiveness with studies?

Would it not be in the interest not only of those who are ill and sometimes dying, but also in the interest of the economy and politics, to put together an intelligent mixture of different methods of healing, which would improve people's health and make their immune system more efficient, so that an infection with SARS-CoV-2 would take its course with no symptoms altogether or only with mild ones?

TCM's greatest strength is prevention. In ancient China, barefoot doctors traveled from village to village and gave those who had particular ailments physical and breathing exercises relevant to the individual case, guidelines for nutrition based on the Five Elements, herbal mixtures, and acupuncture points for cupping and moxibustion. The aim was that chronic diseases wouldn't even begin to develop.

If the majority of the people remained healthy, doctors were welcome to visit again and receive their payment. If many got ill, they would no longer be allowed to enter the village.

The Daoist system identifies seven steps of healing — a list of priorities for prevention and healing.

The seven steps of healing

The highest step of healing is the training of mindfulness toward the inside and the outside using meditation. Our mind formats how we perceive the world and what we think about the world. This is the foundation of our decisions as to what we do and don't do. Our health and vitality are not only determined by our life habits, by exercise and nutrition, and by the balance of activity and rest but also by our mental attitude with regard to living out of our feelings. If we don't follow our own inner voice when it comes to the demands of our social environment, this can manifest itself in the form of a reduction in the courage with which we face life and also in our health.

In order to prevent diseases, or even better, to avoid them by prevention, for Daoism, as in many other cultures, the most important foundation of healing was the purification of the spirit, the recognition of error and changes to one's own way of living. For most illnesses are only the tip of the iceberg of unhealthy living. "Unhealthy" not only refers to the physical but also the emotional and mental sphere of our lives — how we express our feelings and how and what we think all day long. In this book, the questions about the criteria of the Five Elements serve the purpose of gaining an overview of what connects the physical, the emotional, and the mental.

The second step of Daoist healing is the conscious use of the breath. Breathing connects different levels within us, even if we are not aware of this most of the time. Our breathing not only keeps our life processes going on a physical level, but it is also firmly connected with our feelings and our awareness. Each sentiment and every form of behavior is related to a particular quality of breathing, a particular rhythm, a particular depth and frequency of breathing. As feelings and thoughts are so closely connected with our breathing, it suggests itself to influence our feelings and thoughts by our breathing. This can be done in two different ways:

first by bringing feelings and thoughts that are "all over the place" through the breathing techniques of Pranayama or Vipassana under control and second by using certain breathing techniques to set free feelings and thoughts from the subconscious which have played a part in the development of lack of vitality or diseases. This is of importance insofar as Traditional Chinese Medicine is in essence psychosomatic, i.e. based on the interaction between body and soul, and in most cases, the approach to treatment is psychological. Here the traditional teaching about the Five Elements is of great importance.

In Daoist Chinese medicine, movement is the third step of healing — even before nutrition, herbal medicine, acupressure, and acupuncture.

Our animal organism has developed over millions of years in movement. Human beings were hunter-gatherers for almost a million years: roaming around in extreme cold or heat, gathering firewood or collecting fruit, and hunting. And in contrast to that, periods of deep rest, hunter-gatherers had a lot of time on their hands when there was nothing to do.

Over the past 10,000 years, the overwhelming majority of human beings have become settled. As farmers and tradespeople, they became the recipients of orders, with priests, warriors, noblemen, and kings giving the orders. And still the working population had to move a lot.

Since the Industrial Revolution in the nineteenth century, humanity has created machines, which saved workers and craftspeople much physical strain, and vehicles, which made it possible to move around without much movement of muscles.

Our organism is no longer experiencing the extent of movement with which it originally developed. Although with the help of advanced and technologically highly developed medicine we are able to treat many diseases well and thus life expectancy is higher than ever before, human beings are much more susceptible to diseases than before and much more helpless without this medicine. We are much more dependent on this medicine than our ancestors. When medicine has not yet developed a vaccination for a new virus, the large majority of human beings fall into expectant rigidity like a rabbit facing a snake. It is as if we as humanity would not exist if our organism had not for a million years been able to cope with a wide range of viruses and bacteria.

Sufficient movement is one of the pillars of health and a felt quality of life. The path to an intensive care grave for those who are no longer able to go walking for a few days or jump into the air for joy is already paved with pills. At present, only about 14% of the population of Europe move sufficiently so that mental and emotional stress can be reduced and muscles can become strong and supple, organs be full of vitality, and the immune system be well functioning.

The first three steps of healing do not even require an externally administered substance. We can observe our spirit and our breath and practice different forms of breathing and movement, even when no nourishment is available. In his book *Autobiography of a Yogi* (1946), Paramahansa Yogananda (1893–1952) describes his encounters with holy men and saints of India at the beginning of the twentieth century whose *siddhis* (material, paranormal, or supernatural powers and abilities that are the result of vegetarian food, frequent fasting, meditation, and yoga) exceed the imagination of modern human beings whose mind is overflowing with mostly mindless information from their smartphones. The book has sold over four million copies and changed the lives of millions. It also changed my life when I read it at the age of 17 because it showed me that there is a transcendent world that has other laws than our normal conception of reality. That's why, in a van with four friends, I drove to India at the age of 17 and later spent three years learning in India and Sri Lanka about that transcendent world.

The fourth step of healing is nutrition. We are talking here about substances administered externally, ranging from those of a fine texture to those of a rough texture.

The substance of the finest texture we can ingest is homeopathic medicine. Then there are trace elements, minerals, and vitamins. Among the substances that can be most effective even if administered in relatively low concentration are healing herbs and medicaments — many medicaments were originally derived from herbal medicine, and others were developed in pharmaceutic research without an original pattern in nature. Foods with more textured substrates are proteins, fats, and carbohydrates. As we live in a more materialistic society (a society where material goods are valued more highly than the spirit or the soul), correct nutrition is regarded as being of higher value than the other steps of healing. Consequently, there are thousands of doctrines about the right way to feed ourselves well.

The fifth step of healing is acupressure and stimulation of acupuncture points by tuning forks of various frequencies. Among the diverse forms of TCM are acupressure and meridian massage, by which flow of the Qì in the meridians can be stimulated more effectively than with acupuncture.

Acupressure, meridian massage, Shiatsu, and different forms of deep bodywork like Shén Dào and Rolfing increase the permeability of the tissue for the Qì and thus are able to balance fullness and emptiness in the different meridians. Only when the Qì flows sufficiently in the meridians can it be guided by the acupuncture needle in a more targeted and effective way.

As with touch (acupressure), heating (Moxa), and needling (acupuncture), we can use sound vibrations applied by tuning forks to work on the organism via the energy guiding points on the surface of the body and thus strengthen vitality and improve health. In most cases, acupressure works more strongly on the psyche and speaks to the image world of the soul, while acupuncture works better in the healing of persistent symptoms and specific diseases — and sound frequencies enable the essence of a person to vibrate and thus to come to the surface.

For a more extensive effect, we can use sound bowls, for a more specifically defined effect tuning forks which are set on the points selected by TCM diagnosis.

Over the last 10 years, I have observed and studied the effect of frequencies which the Swiss mathematician and musicologist Hans Cousto describes in his book *The Cosmic Octave: Origin of Harmony*. Using the frequencies calculated by him and tuning forks based on them, I was able to observe on myself and many others a wide range of healing effects. I created a method — stimulating the acupuncture points with tuning forks — and have been teaching it in the past eight years.

The sixth step of healing are "stabbing and burning": acupuncture and moxibustion. The seventh step is surgery.

If we follow the first steps, the subsequent ones are more effective. With the practice of differentiated breathing techniques and specific movement exercises such as meridian Qì Gong focusing on the diseased organ, herbal medicine, acupressure, and acupuncture are effective within a shorter space of time and to a larger extent.

I described the Seven Steps of Healing of Daoist Chinese Medicine in two other books that have not been translated to English yet (*Gesund trotz Corona: Der Weg zum schlauen Immunsystem = Health Despite Corona: The Path to a Clever Immune System*, and *Das Tao der Akupressur und Akupunktur = The Dào of Acupressure and Acupuncture*).

The Healing Dào focuses on understanding the system of the Five Elements, specifically on breathing as the second step of healing in the chapter on metal, and on movement (specifically the Qì Gong Exercises for each of the Twelve Organs) as the third step of healing.

The most important measures for keeping the mainly seated *Homo urbanus* are sufficient movement and balanced eating.

In my book *The Dào of Acupressure and Acupuncture* (forthcoming from World Scientific Publishing), I describe the 361 classical points with the psychosomatic indications for acupressure and acupuncture in detail.

The year of the metal rat

The 25th of January 2020 was the beginning of the Year of the Metal Rat. The Rat is the first of the twelve signs of the classical Chinese zodiac, the beginning of the 12-year cycle.

It is a year of new beginnings, say the Chinese astrologers, and new beginnings involve birth pangs and painful learning processes. Once again this was very exact. The economic, political, and social changes affected by the pandemic will shape the coming 12 years. In the economy, many big investors, such as the Rockefeller Brothers Fund, have taken a lot of money out of oil and coal and invested it in sustainable parts of the economy. The Chinese element Metal stands for following abstract principles and demands. In the coming years, the ideology of slowing down climate change will take shape and all parts of the economy will be reassessed.

In politics and society, camera surveillance and contact tracing will continue to be developed, both overtly and covertly. Health apps are a further milestone on the road of social control by the state. Rats are intelligent and they like to control.

Metaphorically, the Year of the Metal Rat bore the dominance of the injection needle (which is made of metal) above other medical systems of the world (with disastrous effects on the health of at least a billion people in Europe, the US, and Canada) and led in 2022 to the first war in Europe since the Yugoslav wars (1991–2001) — artillery, missiles and tanks are made of metal.

The COVID-19 pandemic has shown strong government control often leading to the restriction of fundamental human rights. The pharmaceutical industry managed with the assistance of the WHO to create the myth that *only* vaccination can help to end the pandemic. Governments (especially in Europe and Canada) followed this myth with conviction and most media stopped doing proper investigations with the result that they frequently became a propaganda tool of the pharmaceutical industry. I saw that within a few months, the media were behaving like the *Prawda* in the Soviet Union, or like the Russian media nowadays.

At least a million videos of scientists, doctors, biologists, pharmacists, and various authors have been deleted by YouTube (who has the power to order this?), articles expressing a varying view were prevented from being published, and alternative medicine and medicaments were ignored, ridiculed, or even prohibited. Doctors who treated COVID-19 with Ivermectin lost their license. People who were not vaccinated were considered second-class citizens and often lost their jobs and their friends. There was strong control and restriction of free mobility, meeting other people, crossing borders and traveling, and suppression of freedom of opinion. Alternative channels for exchange of views and information like Telegram came under heavy criticism for the distribution of "fake news" or "disinformation." In Brazil, Telegram channels were closed by court order. But who decides what is true or false when it comes to information? It seems we are going back to general state control akin to the era of the Cold War.

In the Russian war against Ukraine, we can see to what the official media channels in Russia deny the war or show a distorted image of what is happening in Ukraine. The Western media judge and flagellate the Russian media restrictions — without noticing and admitting that they only have been allowing one-sided views on the pandemic themselves for the last two years. It is always easier to see faults in other people than to acknowledge our own. The main impetus of Putin to attack Ukraine seems to be to regain control of this neighboring country so that it does not become too democratic, does not come too much under the influence of Western lifestyles and ideas, and finally does not become too wealthy — showing a sharp contrast to the poverty of many Russians, developing some wealth in only eight years since the Maidan Revolution in 2014. Since 2020, the Chinese government has also regained control of big Chinese corporations and powerful social media, thus also restricting the growth of Western cultural habits.

These three examples show the bias of the element Metal to control, and not to let things flow which is the essence of the element Water, the next element in the cycle. The emotional spectrum of the element Metal ranges from hope and optimism to depression and despair, from open connectedness with the world to self-opinionatedness, dogmatism, and fanaticism, and these basic polarities of sentiment and spirit are the basic tone of the coming years in the light of progressing climate change.

In Chinese Five-Element thinking, 2008 was the Year of the Earth Rat. The element Earth stands for matter, social security, and confidence in society. 2008 was the beginning of a global financial crisis which then with the national indebtedness of Greece turned into the Euro crisis. 2008 was likewise a year of disruption that shaped the coming years. Many citizens lost their confidence in the state for good, as they saw that the state was more prone to protect its banks and the bonuses of those in high finance than its own citizens.

Practical Solutions

We can see that we can apply Five-Element thinking to economy and politics as well as to health and disease. It is a tool to understand the complexities of the outer and the inner world.

Five-Element thinking changed my view of the world. In the beginning, this change is subtle. It is only a colorful set of ideas. If you go on seeing the phenomena of the world as an interplay of forces of nature, it is a good base to understand ecology and the importance to preserve nature.

Human beings today are ten thousand times more concerned with human rights and affairs than with animal and plant rights and the right of nature to persist in an original and undisturbed context. Mankind got into the frenzy to exploit anything on the planet. It followed the saying "Be fruitful and multiply, and replenish the earth and subdue it" from the biblical book Genesis to a much greater extent than many ecosystems can bear.

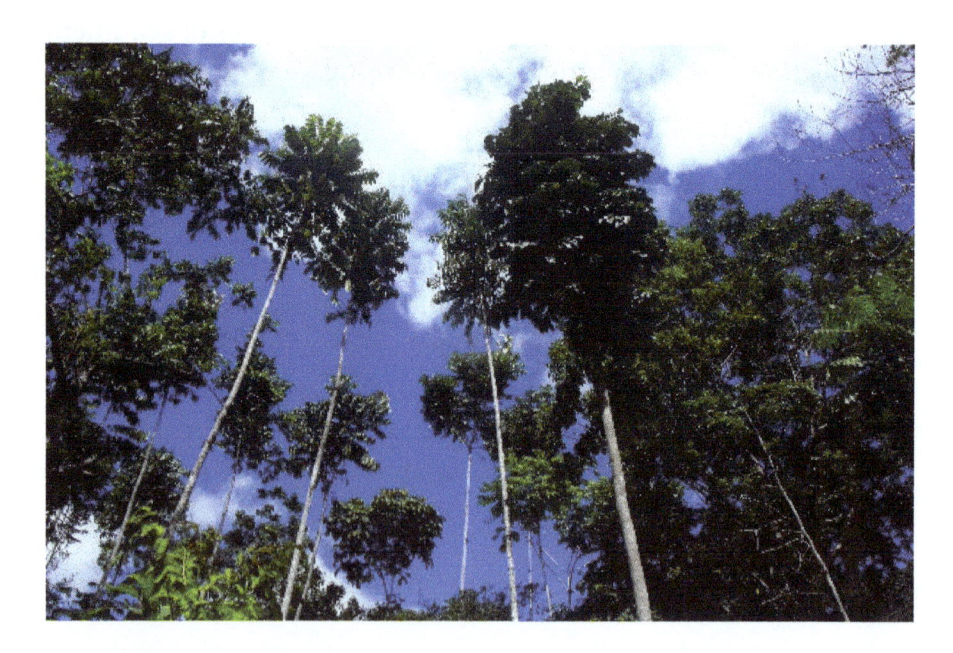

In the long run, Five-Element thinking might change not only the way you see things but also the way you act.

In 2009, I stepped upon a land on the side of a small river in the Brazilian rainforest. Part of it had been burnt down in the 1990s to raise cattle. Part of it remained primarily rainforest with huge trees and a high biodiversity. The soil was not good enough to feed cattle, thus the idea was abandoned and a secondary forest, called *capoeira*, started to grow. The *capoeira* has less biodiversity and needs a century to become a thick forest that contains enough moisture to give shelter to many plants and animals during dry season. I like the land and the river, and thus I go there once a year to plant a hundred trees in the *capoeira* to help biodiversity, mostly rare species, trees that have red, orange, or yellow flowers, trees that one day might be 30 or even 50 meters high. Mahogany trees that I planted 10 years ago are now 10 meters high. It's not a plantation for money; it's a plantation for beauty.

As in my youth, I was more an intellectual and musician than a nature lover, I have the suspicion that Five-Element thinking over the years eased my way to spending part of my time now in the forest admiring trees, planting trees, and caring for nature.

Classification by the Five Elements

	Wood	Fire	Earth	Metal	Water
Yin/Yáng	Young Yáng	Old Yáng	Neutral	Young Yin	Old Yin
Movement	Expansion	Vertically upward	Horizontal here and there	Concentration	Gravitation
Direction	East	South	Middle	West	North
Season	Spring	Summer	Late summer	Fall	Winter
Weather	Windy	Hot	Humid	Dry	Cold
Energetic Character	Tepid, mild, warm	Steaming hot	Neutralizing	Cooling	Bitter cold and frozen
Time of Day	Morning	Midday	Afternoon	Evening	Night
Life Cycle	Birth and growth	Blossoming	Ripening and change	Late ripening and decline	Stagnation and downfall
Use of the Energy to	Sprout	Blossom	Ripen	Harvest	Store
The Five Zàng	Liver	Heart	Spleen/Pancreas	Lungs	Kidneys
The Five Fu	Gallbladder	Small Intestine	Stomach	Large Intestine	Bladder
Tissue	Muscles and tendons	Blood vessels	Connecting tissue	Skin	Bones and bone marrow
Sensory Organs	Eyes	Tongue	Mouth	Nose	Ears

(Continued)

(Continued)

	Wood	Fire	Earth	Metal	Water
The Five Senses	Seeing	Speaking	Touching	Tasting and smelling	Hearing
Bodily Fluid	Tears	Perspiration	Saliva and lymph	Mucus	Urine
Expression of Energy	Nails	Complexion	Lips	Body hair	Hair (head)
Color	Green	Red	Yellow and brown	White	Blue and black
Complexion When Ill	Light green, olive	Mixture of red and white	Yellowish	Pale	Dirty gray, dark brown
Smell When Ill	Sour, rancid	Burned, singed	Unpleasantly sweet	Smokey, spoiled, rotten, fishy	Decayed
Behavior When Stressed	Control	Sadness and worry	Stubborn, rigid, belching	Denial, coughing	Shaking
Emotion	Courage, irritability, anger, rage	Joy, humor, extraversion, chattiness, pride	Compassion, empathy, caring, melancholy, worrying	Withdrawal, sadness, grief	Lust, awe, anxiety, fear
Tone of Voice	Loud shouting	Laughing, giggling	Melodic singing	Whining	Groaning, deep voice
Predominant Temperament	Choleric	Sanguine, joyful	Phlegmatic, compulsive	Melancholic, discouraged	Fearful, paranoid
Elemental Spirit	*Hún:* Soul, vision, inspiration	*Shén:* Consciousness, love	*Yì:* Intellect, practical intelligence	*Po:* Instinct	*Zhì:* Will to live, libido
Functions of the Elemental Spirit	Plans and decisions, organization	Expression, leadership, consciousness	Intellect, reflection, memory	Concentration, abstract and analytical thinking	Awe, awareness, meditation

(Continued)

	Wood	Fire	Earth	Metal	Water
Form of Energy	Spiritual	Psychological	Physical	Vital	Ancestral
Form of Therapy to Strengthen Elements	Sports, martial arts, bioenergetics	Moxibustion, acupuncture, psychotherapy	Diet, massage, bodywork, singing	Breathing exercises, pranayama, aromatherapy	Meditation, vipassana, hypnotherapy
Dream Analysis (A Few Examples)	Forrest, trees, fighting, battles	Fire, laughter, crowds	Singing, music, eating, drinking	Flying, sky, white objects	Water, ocean ships, drowning
Flavor	Sour	Bitter	Sweet	Spicy	Salty
Grain	Wheat, rye	Corn	Millet	Rice, oats	Beans
Fruits	Plums, berries	Apricots	Dates	Peaches	Grapes
Preparation	Steam	Eat raw	Stew, roast	Bake	Grill
Tonifying	Licorice	Ginseng	Orange peel	Cayenne	Marshmallow
Sedating	Sage	Caraway	Basil	Ginger, garlic	Parsley
Astrological Yáng-Animal	Tiger	Horse	Ox, dragon	Monkey	Bear
Astrological Yin-Animal	Rabbit	Snake	Dog, sheep	Rooster	Rat
Yáng-Numbers	3	7	5	9	1
Yin-Numbers	8	2	10	4	6

Bibliography

Arvay, C. *The Biophilia Effect: A Spiritual and Scientific Exploration of the Healing Bond between Humans and Nature*. Sounds True, 2018.

Capra, F. *The Tao of Physics*. Shambhala Publications, 2010.

Harari, Y. N. *Sapiens: A Brief History of Humankind*. Signal, 2014.

Hof, W. *The Wim Hof Method: Activate Your Full Human Potential*. Sounds True, 2022.

Lorenz, K. *On Aggression, Harcourt*. Brace & World, 1966.

Lowen, A. *Bioenergetics. Coward*, McCann & Geoghegan, 1975.

Nestor, J. *Breath — The New Science of a Lost Art*. Penguin Publishing Group, 2020.

Osho. *When the Shoe fits – Talks on Chuang Tzu*. Rajneesh Foundation, 1981.

Osho. *Tao: The Three Treasures, Volume One: Talks on Fragments from the Tao Te Ching by Lao Tzu*. Rajneesh Foundation, 1983.

Osho. *Tantra: The Supreme Understanding*. Osho International Foundation, 2009.

Osho. *The Book of the Secrets: 112 Meditations to Discover the Mystery*. Osho International Foundation, 2010.

Osho. *The Heart Sutra — Becoming a Buddha through Meditation*. Osho International Foundation, 2014.

Paech, N. *Liberation from Excess: The Road to a Post-Growth Economy*. Oekom, 2012.

Rosling, H. *Factfulness: Ten Reasons We're Wrong about the World — And Why Things are Better than you Think*. Sceptre, 2018.

Seem, M., Kaplan, J. *Bodymind Energetics*. Simon & Schuster, 1987.

Sun-Tzu. *The Art of War*. Penguin Classics, 2008.

Wohlleben, P. *The Hidden Life of Trees - What They Feel, How They Communicate*. Greystone Books, 2016.

Index

A
abundance, 66, 68–69
adrenal glands, 108–109
aggression, 18–19, 21, 26–27, 128
aggressive behavior, 34
allergies, 71, 73
Ancestral Energy, 11, 104
anger, 18–21, 27, 33, 127
angina pectoris, 49
annoyance, 19
anxiety, 110
apathy, 20
appendix, 71
auto-aggressive diseases, 24
auto-immune diseases, 21, 73
awareness, 44

B
bitterness, 20
blood, 72
blood pressure, 109
blood vessels, 46
B-lymphocytes, 73
body temperature, 50
bone marrow, 72, 106
brain, 107
breasts, 73
breath, 87–88
buzzing in the ears, 109, 126

C
cheerfulness, 131
chronic colds, 126
circulatory problems, 49
circulatory system, 46, 109
compulsive behavior, 70
concentration, 86, 91
confusion, 26
consciousness, 52
constipation, 73
criticism, 128

D
Dào, 13
deafness, 109
depression, 20–21, 25, 127, 131
diarrhea, 73, 126
digestion, 50, 71
duodenum, 7

E
edema, 73
element, 13
empathy, 128
endocrine system, 108
enthusiasm, 131
epilepsy, 23–24, 49
erythrocytes, 72

F
fear, 109–110, 128
fertility, 66–67, 73–74
Fire-Kidney, 108
fixed ideas, 70
frustration, 20
Fu, 8
fury, 19

G
gastritis, 73
genetic constitution, 105
glands, 108
growth, 22–23, 40

H
hatred, 21
heart attacks, 46
heart pains, 49
high blood pressure, 24, 46
hormones, 108
hypochondriac, 24
hysteria, 49, 131

I
immune deficiencies, 73
immune system, 72–73
impatience, 127
infertility, 73
inflammation of the middle ear, 109
insomnia, 49, 131
irritability, 19, 127

J
joy, 44, 50, 127–128, 131

L
large intestine, 88
laughter, 44
loneliness, 128
love, 29, 46
lungs, 87–88
Luò vessels, 9
lymphatic vessels, 71, 73
lymph glands, 7
lymph nodes, 71–73
lymphocytes, 72

M
mania, 131
manic depression, 49
martial arts, 35
meditation, 110
melancholy, 128
menstrual cycle, 73
menstrual disorders, 24
menstrual problems, 71, 73
middle-ear infections, 126
migraine headaches, 24
motivation, 48

N
nervousness, 49
nervous system, 107

O
obsessions, 70
oral character, 67

P
pancreas, 7, 71–72
pancreatitis, 73

panic attacks, 110
paranoia, 110
pituitary gland, 108
pneumonia, 126
Po, 90
pregnancy, 73

R
rage, 19–20
rational intellect, 69
red bone marrow, 71–73
reflection, 70
resignation, 20, 21
reticulo-endothelial system (RES), 71–72
revelry, 131

S
sadness, 89, 128, 132
schizophrenia, 23
security, 68–69
self-assurance, 67
self-pity, 67
serenity, 131
sexuality, 27, 48, 50
Shén, 45
Shí, 11
skin, 90
skin diseases, 73, 90
small intestine, 7
speech disorders, 48–49
spirituality, 131
spleen, 7, 72–73
stomach, 7

stomach ulcers, 71
suicide, 25
sympathy, 128

T
tachycardia, 49
terror, 110
thymus, 71, 108
thyroid, 108
tiredness, 25
T-lymphocytes, 73
tonsils, 7, 71
tooth decay, 126

V
vision, 26

W
Water-Kidney, 108
wealth, 69
Wèi Qì, 11
worrying, 69

X
Xu, 11

Y
Yáng-Kidney, 47, 108–109
Yin-Kidney, 108
Yong Qì, 11

Z
Zàng, 8
Zong Qì, 11

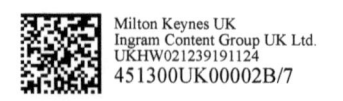